Obstetrics and Gynecology:

The Clinical Core

Obstetrics and Gynecology:

The Clinical Core

RALPH M. WYNN, M.D.
Professor and Head, Department of Obstetrics and Gynecology
The University of Arkansas
College of Medicine, Little Rock, Arkansas

SECOND EDITION

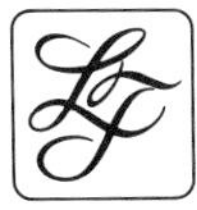

LEA & FEBIGER · 1979 · PHILADELPHIA

First Edition 1974
Reprinted 1975

Library of Congress Cataloging in Publication Data

Wynn, Ralph M
Obstetrics and gynecology.
Includes index.
1. Obstetrics. 2. Gynecology. I. Title.
RG101.W96 1979 618 78-12821
ISBN 0-8121-0658-X

Published in Great Britain by Henry Kimpton Publishers, London
Printed in the United States of America

Print Number 3 2 1

To my medical students and residents,
without whose enthusiastic support this volume
would not have been written

Preface

EDUCATION may be defined as planned change in behavior of the student over a period of time. Medical educators, in common with their colleagues in other fields, must therefore select experiences and teach them as rapidly and efficiently as possible to the level of performance described as acceptable behavior. The planning of medical curricula, including the process of selection, design, and sequential arrangement of instructional units, requires a rationale and thus cannot be left to chance.

About 10 years ago the American Association of Obstetricians and Gynecologists Foundation embarked on its venture of sponsoring a subcommittee to plan a core curriculum in obstetrics and gynecology that might, with local modifications, be tested in schools of medicine throughout the United States. Faculty worked closely with professional educators to construct a curriculum based on four educational principles: development of objectives, preparation of an entry test, construction of a set of learning activities, and formulation of procedures for evaluation of the results.

A core curriculum defines the criteria for minimal competence required of all medical students. It provides at least three major advantages in the educational process. First, it reduces the amount of purely factual material to be learned. Second, it identifies the requisite knowledge and skill for all medical students. Third, it increases the time available for elective studies in the basic or clinical sciences.

The availability of a core curriculum that details the data base frees the teacher from the task of mere dissemination of information and allows him time for influencing attitudes and demonstrating skills. In a modern curriculum the student may proceed at his own rate to accomplish the educational objectives of the core and may devote more time to mastering areas of difficulty. The faster learner may pursue areas in depth or proceed to other areas. The construction of a core curriculum is thus a step toward increased flexibility in the undergraduate medical curriculum. It spells out the *minimal needs of every physician for knowledge and skills in obstetrics and gynecology* and allows time for additional electives or special tracks for students who choose a career in this field.

A good textbook is probably the fastest means of transmitting a large body of knowledge. The skilled reader can control his rate of learning and can read the printed page more rapidly than any lecturer can deliver the same material intelligibly. As self-instructional media and synopses increase in quality and as retrieval of information from handbooks and other reference sources improves, the classic textbook, which struggles in vain to be both instructionally sound and encyclopedic, will gradually disappear. Quite different is the student text based on educational principles. It seldom presents new knowledge. Instead, it offers the available knowledge to the student in a *selective, sequential, simplified* presentation.

Although I have sought the advice of many colleagues and students in the preparation of this book, I accept full responsibility for the selection and arrangement in sequence of the material. I have made extensive use of the valuable publication of the American College of Obstetricians and Gynecologists entitled *Obstetric-Gynecologic Terminology* and have attempted to make the definitions of terms in this text consistent with the recommendations of the Committee of Terminology of the A.C.O.G. wherever possible.

During preparation of this second edition, changes were made on virtually every page of the text. The most extensive revisions occurred in the sections on gynecologic endocrinology, oncology, and particularly control of reproduction. I have attempted to include all essential new information without substantially increasing the size of the book. The largest additions were in basic reproductive biology, which includes sections on gametogenesis, embryology, placental structure and function, and genetics. This change reflects a trend to incorporation of a brief course in basic human reproduction in the curricula of many American medical schools.

Among my colleagues who provided valuable advice in preparation of this edition are, in alphabetical order: Dr. Jack

Bulmash (medical complications), Dr. Leon Chesley (pre-eclampsia), Dr. Timothy Miller (infections), Dr. Thomas Sedlacek (oncology), Dr. Richard Stark (gametogenesis), Dr. Albert Tsai (endocrinology), Dr. Harold Verhage (embryology), Dr. Asuncion Zamora (anesthesiology), and Dr. Lourens Zaneveld (male reproductive biology). Major assistance was provided by several of my former students, who commented from the consumer's point of view during each phase of preparation of this text. Mr. Paul Becton proofread the entire text in both galley and pages and capably assisted in preparation of the index. I am again grateful to Mr. Edward Wickland, Mr. Thomas Colaiezzi, and Ms. Mary Mansor of Lea & Febiger for their efficient and cooperative expedition of all phases of production of this textbook.

RALPH M. WYNN, M.D.

Little Rock, Arkansas

Contents

Notes on the use of this text

The importance of each paragraph is indicated by the presence or absence of vertical lines at the left-hand margin of the text. The information contained in the paragraphs with no vertical lines is the *clinical core*. Because this is the minimal information in obstetrics and gynecology required of all medical students, 100% of it must be mastered. The italicized words provide for a rapid topical review. The material within paragraphs with a single vertical line at the left-hand margin contains additional important elements of the data base that may be included appropriately on undergraduate examinations in obstetrics and gynecology. The material within paragraphs with a double vertical line at the left-hand margin is presented primarily for students who are considering a career in this field.

The core text defines only the data base required for minimal competence in the cognitive domain of obstetrics and gynecology. Detailed information, illustrative material, and references must be sought in standard textbooks, specialized treatises, and periodicals. Audiovisual aids, lectures, conferences, rounds, and clinical experiences with patients are required to achieve educational objectives in the affective and psychomotor (skills) domains. The basic reproductive biology included in this volume should provide the student with essential information for successful completion of an entry test to a clerkship in obstetrics and gynecology.

Obstetrics and Gynecology:

The Clinical Core

UNIT I

History and Physical Examination

The Gynecologic and Obstetric History

The patient's *age* is a most important factor in the evaluation of gynecologic signs and symptoms. For example, in the *child-bearing* age the most important causes of *uterine bleeding* are associated with disorders of *reproduction*. In *postmenopausal* women, *carcinomas* of the genital tract figure prominently in differential diagnosis, whereas in *adolescent* girls the cause of abnormal uterine bleeding is much more likely to be *endocrine*.

Gravidity is synonymous with pregnancy and a *gravida* is a pregnant woman. A *primigravida*, or gravida 1, is a woman who is pregnant for the first time. A *secundigravida* is a woman in her second pregnancy. A *multigravida* is a pregnant woman who has been pregnant *several times*. The numeric designation of gravidity is not altered by *plural gestation*. For example, a patient who is pregnant for the first time with *twins* is *gravida 1*, and she becomes gravida 2 during her second pregnancy.

Parity is the state of having given birth to an infant weighing *500* g or more, alive or dead. When the weight of the infant is not known, an estimated gestational length of *20 weeks* or more, calculated from the first day of the last menstrual period, may be used to establish parity. For purposes of defining parity, *plural gestations* are counted the *same as singleton* pregnancies.

A *primipara* is a woman who has given birth for the first time to an infant or infants, alive or dead, weighing 500 g or more. A primigravida is often incorrectly designated a primipara. A *multipara* is a woman who has given birth two or more times to an infant or infants weighing 500 g or more, alive or dead. The designation *"grand" multipara* is often applied to a woman who has given birth seven or more times to an infant or infants weighing 500 g or more.

According to one common method of summarizing the obstetric history, the number of *abortions* is listed separately. For example, a woman who has had two term pregnancies, one of which was a twin pregnancy, and one abortion, and is now pregnant would be *gravida 4, para 2, ab 1*. Abortions should be recorded as *spontaneous* or *induced* (medically indicated or elective).

An alternative scheme for recording obstetric data uses four digits. The first refers to the number of *term* pregnancies, the second to the number of *premature* deliveries, the third to the number of *abortions*, and the fourth to the number of *living children*. The history of the gravida 4, para 2, ab 1 just described may be abbreviated in the four digit system as 2-0-1-3. A woman whose only pregnancy terminated in premature quintuplets, all of whom survived, would be designated para 0-1-0-5.

A *parturient* is a woman in the process of giving birth. A *puerpera* is a woman who has given birth during the preceding 42 days.

The *chief complaint* is the basic reason that the patient is seeking medical attention. In arriving at a diagnosis, it is often profitable to use the *patient's own words* in describing her chief complaint. Clinical acumen and experience are often required to discern the *real reason* behind the alleged chief complaint. For example, sexual incompatibility may often be presented as vulvar pruritus, or a fear of cancer may be expressed as concern over a trivial vaginal discharge.

The *present illness* should be described in detail. *Listening* to the patient carefully *without undue direction* of the questioning will usually provide most of the pertinent diagnostic information. In obtaining a gynecologic history, details of the following signs and symptoms should be elicited: changes or abnormalities in *uterine bleeding; pain* in the lower abdomen, flank, vagina, or external genitalia; a *lesion* on the *external genitalia* or a palpable *mass* in the *pelvis;* a change in the quality or quantity of *vaginal discharge;* changes in *gastrointestinal* or *urinary habits; protrusion* of the *vaginal wall;* and *infertility.*

When the major complaint involves a change or abnormality in *uterine bleeding*, a *detailed menstrual history* should be obtained at this point. When the chief complaint and present illness are not related primarily to vaginal bleeding, an abbreviated menstrual history should be recorded after the present illness.

The menstrual history should include the age of onset of menstrual periods (*menarche*), the *interval* between the periods, the *duration* of flow, the *amount* of flow as measured by the number of pads or tampons used, the date of the *last normal menstrual period* (LNMP), and the date of the *preceding* menstrual period (PMP). A formula for recording menarche, interval between periods in days, and duration of flow in days is exemplified by *14 × 28 × 4,* which indicates that menarche occurred at age 14, the first day of the period follows the first day of the preceding period by 28 days, and the duration of flow is 4 days. *Dysmenorrhea* (painful periods) and signs and symptoms of *premenstrual tension* should be recorded as part of the menstrual history.

Primary dysmenorrhea (essential, or functional, dysmenorrhea) is menstrual pain in the absence of a recognized pelvic lesion (p. 223). *Secondary dysmenorrhea* is menstrual pain caused by demonstrable pelvic disease.

Premenstrual tension is a condition characterized by increased nervousness, irritability, emotional instability, depression, frequent headaches, and edema. The syndrome may include painful swelling of the breasts, abdominal bloating, nausea, vomiting, fatigue, and a variety of other complaints. Premenstrual tension occurs during the 7 to 10 days preceding menstruation and usually disappears a few hours after the onset of menstrual flow (p. 224).

In older women, the date of the last menstrual period (*menopause*) and a history of associated symptoms such as hot flashes and sweating should be elicited. The menopause strictly refers to the cessation of menstrual function, whereas the *climacteric* is the period of a woman's life characterized by cessation of menses as well as vasomotor changes and a variety of endocrine, somatic, and psychic readjustments (p. 217).

In an adult woman the relation of changes in uterine bleeding to use of *exogenous hormones* including *oral contraceptives* and *postmenopausal replacement* should be clarified. Changes in menstrual patterns should be distinguished from uterine bleeding unrelated to the menses.

Menorrhagia is excessive (*hypermenorrhea*) or prolonged menstrual bleeding, whereas *metrorrhagia* is irregular acyclic uterine bleeding. *Menometrorrhagia* is irregular or excessive uterine bleeding during menstruation as well as between menstrual periods. Menometrorrhagia may be a sign of a variety of diseases and is not a diagnostic entity.

Hypomenorrhea is a diminution in the amount of flow or a shortening of the duration of menstruation. *Oligomenorrhea* is a reduction of the frequency of menstruation, in which the interval between the cycles is longer than 38 days but less than three months. The opposite of oligomenorrhea is *polymenorrhea,* which is abnormally frequent menstruation.

Abnormalities of bleeding confined to the *menses* are often of *endocrine* origin, whereas *intermenstrual* bleeding suggests other lesions including benign and malignant *neoplasms.* Bleeding after *contact* (intercourse or douching) should always suggest a malignant lesion.

Pain should be described in terms of *location, onset,* and *character.* The history should note whether the pain is diffuse or localized, sharp or dull, constant or intermittent, mild or severe; whether it is abdominal, pelvic, vaginal, or lumbar; and whether it *radiates* to the thighs or is *referred* to the shoulder. Pain referred to the low back or buttocks is often associated with diseases of the cervix, urethra, or lower portions of the bladder and rectum. Pain localized to the lower abdomen may arise from the uterus or vagina. Adnexal pain is usually referred to the lower abdominal quadrants and often radiates down the medial aspect of the thigh. Dysmenorrhea and dyspareunia should be recorded at this point. The pain should be described as acute or chronic and its onset as sudden or gradual. If a *precipitating event* is ascertained, it should be recorded along with associated signs and symptoms of *urinary tract* or *gastrointestinal disease,* such as nausea, vomiting, dysuria, chills, and fever. The *sequence* of events preceding and following the onset of pain should be meticulously described and recorded chronologically. Any factors that ameliorate or aggravate the discomfort should be noted.

In describing *vaginal discharge,* the relation to *menses* and *coitus* and the *response* to *therapy* should be noted. It must be recognized that vaginal discharge may stem from a primary lesion of the *vulva, cervix,* or *corpus.*

In obtaining a history of *urinary incontinence* it is necessary to differentiate *stress incontinence* (loss of urine upon increase in intraabdominal pressure, as in straining and coughing) from *frequency* and *urgency* with dribbling unrelated to stress and from *true incontinence,* which is a more or less constant loss of urine. In eliciting a history of *fecal incontinence,* obstetric injuries and gynecologic procedures of possible etiologic importance must be noted.

Various complaints referable to *pelvic relaxation* are common in parous women. The *history* is of paramount importance in these patients because treatment is based more on symptoms than on purely anatomic defects.

Tables 1 through 3 are useful guides to recording the obstetric and gynecologic history and physical examination in institutions that employ this conventional method of obtaining these

TABLE 1. Gynecologic and Obstetric History

I. Age and Parity

II. Chief Complaint

III. Present Illness

A. *Bleeding*
1. Change in interval, duration, and amount of menstrual bleeding
2. Intermenstrual bleeding
3. Contact bleeding
4. Postmenopausal bleeding
5. Relation to exogenous steroids

B. *Pain*
1. Location
2. Relation to menses
3. Radiation
4. Character

C. *Mass*
1. Location
2. Time of onset
3. Rate of growth
4. Pain, discomfort, pruritus, discharge, or bleeding
5. Relation to menses

D. *Vaginal discharge*
1. Color, odor, and consistency
2. Onset, duration, and quantity
3. Pain or pruritus

TABLE 1 (*Continued*)

E. *Urinary and gastrointestinal symptoms*
   1. Frequency, urgency, dysuria, urinary incontinence, and hematuria
   2. Diarrhea, constipation, tenesmus, fecal incontinence, rectal bleeding

F. *Protrusion through the vagina*
   1. Sensation of mass falling out
   2. Difficulty in emptying bowel
   3. Stress incontinence of urine
   4. Relaxed vaginal outlet

G. *Infertility*
   1. Female factors (endometrial biopsy; tubal patency test)
   2. Male factors (sperm count)
   3. Reproductive incompatibility (refer to specialist)

IV. Menstrual History

A. *Age of menarche*
B. *Character of early cycles*
C. *Interval between normal periods*
D. *Amount and duration of normal periods*
E. *Associated signs and symptoms*
F. *Last normal menstrual period and previous normal menstrual period*
G. *Premenstrual tension*
H. *Abnormalities of uterine bleeding*
I. *Hypomenorrhea or amenorrhea*
J. *Relation to oral contraceptives*
K. *Menopause*
   1. Date of last menses
   2. Climacteric symptoms

V. Obstetric History

A. *Dates of deliveries*
B. *Lengths of gestations*
C. *Complications during pregnancy (bleeding, headache, edema)*

TABLE 1 (*Continued*)

- D. *Durations of labors*
- E. *Methods of deliveries (spontaneous, forceps, cesarean section)*
- F. *Weight, sex, and condition of each infant at delivery*
- G. *Number and health of children now alive*
- H. *Postpartum complications*
- I. *Abortions*
  1. Spontaneous
  2. Medically indicated
  3. Elective

VI. Contraceptive History

- A. *Type of contraceptive used*
- B. *Duration of use*
- C. *Reason for choice*
- D. *Satisfaction with method*
- E. *Effectiveness of method*
- F. *Undesirable side effects*

VII. Sexual History

- A. *Regularity and type of sexual activity*
- B. *Libido, satisfaction, and orgasm*
- C. *Dyspareunia, frigidity, and other sexual problems such as premature ejaculation*

VIII. Medical History

- A. *Diabetes*
- B. *Hypertension*
- C. *Cardiac disease*
- D. *Renal disease*
- E. *Syphilis*
- F. *Tuberculosis*
- G. *Epilepsy*
- H. *Exposure to rubella*
- I. *Allergies*
- J. *Present medications*

TABLE 1 (*Continued*)

IX. Surgical History

A. *Dates of operations*
B. *Surgeons and hospitals where performed*
C. *Diagnoses*
D. *Results*

X. Family History

A. *Twinning*
B. *Hereditary diseases*

XI. Social History

A. *Tobacco*
B. *Alcohol*
C. *Occupation*
D. *Hobbies and recreational activities*

data. In institutions that use the *problem-oriented record*, the same information must be elicited but is generally recorded in the following four categories: objective data, subjective data, assessment, and plan.

The Gynecologic Examination

Every gynecologic and obstetric examination should be preceded by a review of systems and a general physical with particular attention to *blood pressure, heart, lungs,* and *eye-grounds.* Whenever a patient is examined by a male gynecologist a *female assistant* should remain in attendance. The patient should *void* before pelvic examination except when stress incontinence of urine is to be demonstrated. It is easier to palpate the pelvic organs if the patient's *rectum* is *empty.* An outline of the examination of breasts and pelvic organs is given in Table 2.

Careful examination of the *breasts* should routinely precede gynecologic examination. *Inspection* and *palpation* may be

TABLE 2. Gynecologic Examination

I. Breasts
   A. *Inflammatory lesions*
   B. *Symmetry*
   C. *Masses*
      1. Cystic or solid
      2. Fixation to overlying skin
      3. Retraction of skin
   D. *Discharge from nipple*
   E. *Tenderness*
   F. *Lymphadenopathy*
      1. Axillary
      2. Supraclavicular

II. Abdomen
   A. *Masses and organomegaly*
   B. *Tenderness*
   C. *Rigidity*
   D. *Bowel sounds*
   E. *Ascites or encapsulated fluid*
   F. *Scars*

III. Pelvic Examination
   A. *External genitalia*
      1. Congenital anomalies
      2. Hair distribution
      3. Size of clitoris
      4. Inflammation, masses, or lesions of Bartholin's glands, urethra, and Skene's glands
      5. Masses, lesions, and ulcerations of the labia majora, labia minora, perineum, and anus
   B. *Vagina*
      1. Partial or complete atresia
      2. Transverse or longitudinal septa
      3. Relaxation of walls
      4. Inflammation and atrophy of the mucosa
      5. Masses or nodularity of the vaginal wall
      6. Discharge

TABLE 2 (*Continued*)

C. *Cytologic examination of cervix and vagina* (*Papanicolaou smear*)

D. *Cervix**

1. Size and shape
2. Configuration of external os
3. Pain on motion
4. Ulcers or masses
5. Color and consistency
6. Contact bleeding

E. *Corpus*

1. Size and configuration
2. Mobility and position
3. Pain on motion

F. *Adnexa*

1. Masses (size and consistency)
2. Pain on motion

G. *Rectovaginal*

1. Nodularity of cul-de-sac
2. Consistency of parametria
3. Rectal or rectovaginal masses
4. Rectal bleeding

*Colposcopy is sometimes included as part of the routine examination of the cervix. Its use in the diagnosis of cervical abnormalities is described on pages 129 and 169.

supplemented by *transillumination*. In cases of doubtful findings, *mammography* (roentgenographic examination to detect cancer or fibrocystic disease) may be employed (p. 160). Inspection and palpation are performed with the patient in *several positions* in order to examine each quadrant of the breast with maximal efficiency. First, the patient sits at the edge of the table with her arms extended upward to optimize examination of the upper quadrants. She then bends forward with her arms extended outward so that the breasts are dependent. *Asymmetry* of the breasts is noted in these positions. Each portion of the breast is palpated to detect size, consistency, tenderness, and fixation of any *masses*. *Bloody discharge* from the nipple should be investigated by a *cytologic smear* as an initial study. Any *retraction* of the skin or nipple and any discrete firm *mass* requires further investigation, usually including *biopsy*. The patient then assumes a *recumbent* position. She first turns on her right side for examination of the inner quadrants of her right breast and the outer quadrants of her left breast. She then turns on her left side for examination of the inner quadrants of the left breast and the outer quadrants of the right breast. The *axilla* is best examined with the tips of the fingers, which should be inserted while the patient's arms are raised. The palpation is carried out after the patient's arm is brought down against the chest wall. After examination of the axilla, an attempt should be made to palpate *supraclavicular nodes*. As the doctor inspects and palpates the patient's breasts he should teach her systematic *self-examination*.

The *abdomen* is next examined by *inspection, palpation, percussion*, and *auscultation* with the patient in the recumbent position. *Scars, striations, diastasis* of the recti, and *hernias* of the abdominal wall should be noted. *Asymmetry* of the abdominal contour suggests an abnormal mass. Large *myomas* are likely to be irregular, whereas a *pregnant uterus* is normally symmetric. An *ovarian cyst* may closely resemble a symmetric myoma. On inspection alone, cystic tumors may be indistinguishable from *ascites*.

Percussion may aid in delimiting the edges of tumors, the height of the urinary bladder, and loops of distended bowel. It may also differentiate the free fluid of ascites from the encapsulated fluid within an ovarian cyst. *Paracentesis* should *not be performed* diagnostically because of the risk of rupturing an ovarian cyst that may be malignant or contain irritating contents that could initiate a chemical peritonitis.

In the case of *ascites* the abdomen is symmetric and there is shifting dullness, dullness in the flanks, and tympany in the anterior abdomen. With an *ovarian cyst* the upper abdomen is flat, and there is seldom shifting dullness, but there is tympany in the flanks and dullness in the anterior abdomen.

Palpation of the upper abdomen should precede that of the lower abdomen and pelvis. In thin women the lower pole of the *kidney* may normally be palpated. An attempt should be made to feel the lower edges of the *liver* and *spleen*. Tenderness in the *costovertebral angles* should be noted. The *inguinal region* should be palpated to detect hernias and lymphadenopathy. Palpation should begin as far away as possible from areas of tenderness. Persistence of *spasm* after a few moments of gentle depression of the anterior abdominal wall suggests peritoneal irritation. The other major sign of peritonitis is *rebound tenderness.*

For the pelvic examination proper, the patient's feet are placed in *stirrups* and her *buttocks* are brought well *over the edge* of the *table*. Her *knees* should be *separated* as *widely* as possible and the examiner positioned comfortably with a well-focused bright light. The *external genitalia* are examined in the following sequence: clitoris, urethral meatus, Skene's ducts, labia minora and majora including Bartholin's ducts, the perineal body, and the perianal region. *Skene's ducts,* the *urethra,* and *Bartholin's ducts* may be inflamed. In the case of acute *gonorrhea* they may produce a purulent discharge. Bartholin's gland is not normally palpable unless involved in a cyst or abscess and its opening onto the labia is not visible except in the presence of inflammation. The size of the *clitoris* should be noted and inflammation, atrophy, ulcer, or discharge involving the *labia, mons,* and *perineum* recorded. After the labia are separated, the *fourchette* and *hymen* should be examined for evidence of tears or scarring. In the virgin the labia majora are apposed. In the nonvirginal nulliparous woman various degrees of gaping and scarring are normal. In parous women these changes are exaggerated. In older women some degree of labial atrophy is normal. At this point the patient is asked to *bear down* to see whether she loses urine on coughing (*stress incontinence*). Descent of the anterior vaginal wall, posterior vaginal wall, or cervix represents *cystocele, rectocele,* and *uterine prolapse,* respectively.

The systematic examination of the genitalia is now interrupted to obtain a *Papanicolaou smear* of the *vagina* and *cervix*. The cytologic examination is done at this point, *before any lubricant* is used. To minimize discomfort during introduction of the unlubricated speculum, the perineum should be depressed, avoiding contact with the anterior portion of the vagina and the clitoris. For best results in cytologic diagnosis, *bleeding* should be *minimal* and the patient should be instructed to *avoid douching* for the 24 hours preceding examination.

Because the Papanicolaou smear is an integral part of the gynecologic examination, it is described in detail here. Its interpretation in connection with other diagnostic procedures is described on pages 129 and 168.

The vaginal *vault* and the cervical *canal* may be *aspirated* with a glass *pipette* or the external cervical *os* and *portio* may be *scraped* with a *wooden spatula* or rubbed with a *cotton-tipped applicator.* The smear should be *fixed immediately* in equal parts of 95% alcohol and ether or dry-fixed with a commercially available spray. The smear must be labeled carefully, preferably by marking the slide itself with a diamond pencil. The smears are generally stained by the *Papanicolaou method* and examined with the light microscope. Occasionally an acridine orange stain is used preparatory to fluorescent microscopy. *Cytologic screening* is a most important procedure that should be performed as part of the physical examination of any woman over the age of 25 and in even younger patients who are sexually active. *No treatment* of a cervical lesion should be attempted before the results of the cytologic screening are available. Electrocauterization and cryosurgical procedures in particular should be deferred until a diagnosis is obtained.

A smear of material pipetted from the posterior fornix includes squamous cells from the vagina and cervix and glandular cells from the endocervix and endometrium. Carcinoma of the cervix is best detected in a smear obtained from around the external os, whereas a scraping from the lateral vaginal wall is best for hormonal cytodiagnosis. Several "do-it-yourself" kits are available for home use in cancer detection, but there are inherent errors in collection of the specimen. Furthermore, the patient is denied the benefit of a simultaneous pelvic examination. The Papanicolaou smear prepared from a single cervical swab is more than 90% accurate in detecting carcinoma of the cervix, but a single vaginal aspiration is not sufficiently accurate for detection of endometrial carcinoma. The endometrial aspiration smear improves the rate of detection of carcinoma of the corpus, but definitive diagnosis of this lesion requires curettage or, at least, adequate endometrial biopsy.

The Papanicolaou smear may be used to assess the woman's hormonal status as part of the investigation of an endocrine disorder or infertility. The maturation index is the ratio of parabasal to intermediate to superficial cells. For example, a maturation index of 0/20/80 indicates a fair estrogenic effect. The maturation index is normally maximal at the time of ovulation. A maturation index (MI) of 20/75/5, for example, represents a poor estrogenic effect. The karyopyknotic index (KI) is the percentage of superficial cells with deeply pigmented (pyknotic) nuclei. A high karyopyknotic index (greater than 30) is considered to reflect a marked estrogenic effect.

Any *suspicious* lesion on the cervix should be subjected to *biopsy* when first detected (p. 129). The biopsy specimen may be obtained through a *single punch* of a localized lesion or a large mass. *Four-quadrant* punches of a circumoral lesion are much less commonly performed today. Selection of a site for biopsy may be facilitated by Schiller staining (p. 129) or, preferably, by colposcopic examination (p. 129). A *cone biopsy* is never performed as an office procedure (p. 130). Since the Papanicolaou smear is only a screening procedure, histologic confirmation is required before any treatment is initiated. The management of the abnormal Papanicolaou smear is diagrammed on page 169.

Before removal of the speculum the *color* of the cervix is noted. A *bluish* discoloration may be an indication of *pregnancy* or a *large tumor*. The condition of the *external os* may indicate *parity*. The nulliparous cervix has a small circular external os, whereas in the parous woman the os is irregular or transversely lacerated.

The *vagina* itself is often inadequately inspected because the speculum covers a large part of its surface. Nevertheless, to detect vaginal lesions, which are attracting increasingly greater attention, the entire surface of the vagina should be carefully inspected under bright light. The *color* of the mucosa and the condition of the *rugae* should be noted. *Nodularities* and *ulcers* should be described. Any suspicious lesion should be subjected to *biopsy*.

An attempt should be made to identify the etiologic agent in any profuse *vaginal discharge*. Organisms that may be identified on initial examination are *Gonococcus, Candida* (*Monilia*), and *Trichomonas*. Discharge from the urethral meatus, Skene's ducts, Bartholin's ducts, the external cervical os, and the anal crypts may be *gram-stained* and *inoculated* on a *Thayer-Martin* agar plate or another suitable culture medium, to identify *gonococci*. Culture is often performed without charge by local health departments.

Hanging-drop smears for *trichomonads* may be obtained from the urethra, external os, or posterior fornix. The material is suspended in normal saline and examined on a glass slide. The *yeast-like* organisms that cause candidiasis may be recognized if some of the cheesy exudate is suspended in 10% *potassium hydroxide* or *cultured* on a medium such as *Nickerson's*, where they will appear as brown or black colonies within 24 hours.

For the remainder of the *internal examination*, the patient remains in the *lithotomy* position. To effect relaxation of the abdominal wall, the patient is asked to take fast shallow breaths. The *uterus* and *adnexa* are palpated between the internal (vaginal) hand and the external (abdominal) hand during the conventional *bimanual* examination. By depressing the patient's perineum and by resting his elbow on his thigh, the examiner may be able to extend his reach into the vagina. The doctor may find it comfortable to rest one foot on a low stool. At the onset of the internal examination, the *cervix* is located and its size, mobility, and consistency noted. Pain on motion of the cervix should be recorded. The *corpus* should then be palpated between the abdominal hand, which makes downward pressure on it, and the vaginal hand, which pushes the uterus upward. The size, mobility, consistency, position, and shape of the uterus should be recorded.

Physical diagnosis is rendered *difficult* when the patient *fails to relax*, when the examination causes *pain*, when the patient is *obese*, and when the *bladder* or *rectum* is *filled*. The *normal fallopian tube* is *rarely palpable* even under ideal conditions of examination. Before an attempt is made to ascertain the size and consistency of the *ovary*, the position and size of the uterus must be known. If an ovarian enlargement is felt, it is most important to describe whether it is *cystic* or *solid*, or *unilateral* or *bilateral*. Because any solid ovarian mass may represent a *malignant* tumor, the description of any adnexal lesion must be accurately recorded. The size of a pelvic mass should be noted in *centimeters* rather than in terms of fruits, vegetables, or eggs of various birds. It is valuable to accompany the description of abnormal findings by a *drawing* since subsequent management may depend on whether a lesion has regressed, remained the same size, or grown since the last examination.

A normal *ovary* may be felt in a thin cooperative patient by even a relatively inexperienced examiner, but even a distinctly enlarged ovary may not be palpable by an expert in an obese or uncooperative patient. If there is any *doubt* about the presence of an adnexal mass, *consultation* should be obtained because any ovarian enlargement is a potentially serious lesion. The average dimensions of the normal adult ovary are *3.0 × 2.0 × 1.5 cm*, although ovarian size varies considerably during the reproductive period. Any adnexal mass greater in size than the normal ovary should be carefully investigated. For accurate diagnosis of an adnexal mass, the pelvic examination must occasionally be performed under anesthesia, especially in children.

The *rectovaginal* examination should be performed *last* because it is usually the most uncomfortable, but it should *never* be *omitted* from the gynecologic examination. The *parametria* and *uterosacral* ligaments, which may be involved in inflammatory or neoplastic diseases, are palpable only on rectovaginal examination. Lesions detected on rectovaginal palpation include a *high rectocele*, an *enterocele* (p. 150), *endometriosis* (p. 153), and masses on the posterior uterine wall and in the cul-de-sac and rectovaginal septum. Palpation of the parametria is requisite to *clinical staging* of carcinoma of the cervix (p. 170). The middle finger is inserted into the rectum and the index finger into the vagina. The tissues of the *rectovaginal septum* are felt between the two fingers. Moving the fingers laterally from the cervix to the right and left permits systematic palpation of the *parametria*.

Occasionally in children and older virgins, the *rectal* examination is substituted for the vaginal. If the findings are suspicious or inconclusive, examination under *anesthesia* may be required. During rectal examination, attention is directed to hemorrhoids, fistulas, fissures, anorectal polyps and tumors, and condylomas.

An outline of the physical examination of the *obstetric*

patient is presented in Table 3, and further details are supplied on pages 22–37.

TABLE 3. Obstetric Examination

I. Uterine Size
II. Consistency and Shape of the Uterus (early in pregnancy)
III. Presentation and Position of the Fetus
IV. Size and Movements of the Fetus
V. Mobility of the Fetal Head
VI. Consistency, Size, and Engagement of the Head
VII. Presence of Fetal Heart Tones (by stethoscope or Doptone)
VIII. Vaginal Examination to Detect Position, Length, Consistency, and Dilatation of the Cervix
IX. Manual Pelvimetry
X. Papanicolaou Smear on the First Antepartum Visit If the Patient Has Not Had a Cytologic Examination Within the Last 12 Months
XI. Chest Film (PA)
XII. Cervical Culture for Gonorrhea

Blood type
Rubella titer

UNIT II

Normal Obstetrics

Diagnosis of Pregnancy

Diagnosis of pregnancy is made on the basis of *history, physical signs and symptoms,* and *laboratory tests.* The signs of pregnancy are classified as *positive, probable,* or *presumptive.* The history must include an accurate account of the *menses,* the *last normal menstrual period, exposure* to pregnancy, and *contraception.*

Positive signs of pregnancy are not elicited before the second trimester by conventional clinical techniques. They include seeing or feeling *fetal movements* by the examining physician, hearing and counting the *fetal heart rate* separately from the maternal pulse, and *radiologic* or *sonographic* delineation of the *fetus.* Fetal movements can normally be felt by the fifth month. The fetal heart beat can be detected by stethoscope by the eighteenth week and by ultrasound (Doppler principle) by the twelfth week. The fetus can be visualized radiologically by the sixteenth week and a gestational sac may be detected sonographically as early as the fifth week.

Probable signs of pregnancy include enlargement of the abdomen, enlargement of the uterus, a globular change in shape of the uterus, softening of the cervix and the lower uterine segment (the area between cervix and corpus), irregular painless contractions of the uterus (Braxton Hicks contractions), ballottement of the uterus (repercussion of the fetus affer tapping the lower uterine segment), and positive hormonal tests for pregnancy. The hormonal tests, which may be immunologic or biologic, depend essentially on the detection of human chorionic gonadotropin, the level of which is normally highest between the fiftieth and ninetieth days of gestation. Progestin-induced withdrawal bleeding is no longer an acceptable technique to rule out pregnancy. Examination of the cervical mucus in pregnancy will reveal either a beaded (cellular) or an intact fern pattern. An intact fern is not compatible with normal early pregnancy.

Presumptive signs and symptoms of pregnancy include amenorrhea, fullness and tenderness of the breasts, enlargement and darkening of the areola, prominence of sebaceous glands of the areola (Montgomery's tubercles), and secretion of thick yellow fluid (colostrum) from the nipple after the first few months. Additional presumptive symptoms include lassitude, nausea and vomiting (morning sickness), frequency of urination, and quickening (appreciation of fetal movements by the patient after the fourth month). Presumptive physical signs include bluish discoloration of the vagina and cervix, increased pigmentation of the skin, and abdominal striae.

The average duration of human pregnancy is 40 weeks (p. 24). To calculate the estimated date of confinement (EDC), count back three months from the last menstrual period (LMP) and add seven days. For example, if the LMP was March 18, 1979, the EDC is December 25, 1979.

There may be an error of approximately two weeks in calculation of the EDC. About 40% of women will deliver within five days of the EDC and about two thirds within 10 days of the EDC. Because a large number of women experience vaginal bleeding during the first two months of pregnancy (p. 76), erroneous calculation of the EDC is not uncommon.

Biologic tests for pregnancy detect the effects of chorionic gonadotropin (a glycoprotein), including formation of a corpus luteum, ovarian hyperemia, and extrusion of eggs or sperm when the appropriate species receives an injection of human urine containing chorionic gonadotropin (hCG). Immunologic tests are 95% accurate (positive) when the patient is pregnant (5% false-negative rate) and are 98% accurate (negative) when the patient is not pregnant (2% false-positive).

The differential diagnosis of pregnancy includes myomas, ovarian cysts, pseudocyesis (false, or spurious, pregnancy), and hematometra (collection of blood within the uterus). With myomas there is usually no amenorrhea and the uterus is firmer. With ovarian cysts the mass may be felt separate from the uterus. Both myomas and ovarian cysts, however, may coexist with pregnancy. With pseudocyesis, a normal-sized uterus may be palpated under anesthesia. The signs of false pregnancy may occasionally be reversed under hypnosis.

Signs of fetal death include failure of growth or regression in size of the uterus, regression of mammary changes, and disappearance of fetal heart tones and fetal movements. Radiologic signs include collapsed skull bones, exaggerated curvature of the spine, gas in the heart and great vessels, and failure to demonstrate swallowing of amniotic fluid into which a contrast medium has been injected (amniography).

Some of the physical signs in a first pregnancy are different from those in later pregnancies. In a woman pregnant for the first time, the abdominal wall is tenser, the uterus and breasts are firmer, the labia may be apposed, and tags of hymen and vaginal rugae are more obvious. The primigravid cervix is more likely to be conical and closed with a regular circular external os. The vagina of the multipara is wider, the vulva gapes, and the external os is irregular.

In the fourth week of pregnancy the level of hCG is 5000 to 6000 IU/liter of urine. By the eighth to twelfth week it has risen to 300,000 IU/liter. By the twentieth week it is back to 3000 to 4000 IU/liter. False-negative pregnancy tests are more commonly encountered before the sixth week of pregnancy, after the middle of pregnancy, in cases of threatened abortion, and in ectopic pregnancy (p. 80). False-positive tests are encountered with proteinuria and in cases in which any of a variety of drugs has been ingested within 24 hours of the test. False-positive results may also be produced by the high levels of pituitary gonadotropin found in midcycle and after the menopause. Pregnancy can be detected earlier by specific radioimmunoassay or radioreceptor assay for the beta subunit of hCG.

A standard immunologic test involves immunizing rabbits against hCG. The urine to be tested is added to this anti-hCG rabbit serum. Sheep erythrocytes coated with hCG are then added. If hemagglutination takes place, the test is negative and the patient is assumed to be not pregnant. Inhibition of hemagglutination is considered to be a positive test indicating pregnancy. The latex inhibition slide tests are rapid and quite convenient, but are somewhat less sensitive.

■ Maternal Physiology

The average *duration* of human pregnancy is 280 days from the first day of the LMP, or 267 days after ovulation. By the *third lunar month* of gestation, the top of the uterus reaches the *pelvic brim*. By the fourth month it is four fingerbreadths above the symphysis. By the fifth month the top of the uterus is almost at the level of the umbilicus. By the *sixth month* it is *slightly above the umbilicus*. By the seventh month it is three fingerbreadths above the umbilicus. By the eighth month it is three fingerbreadths above the level reached in the seventh month. By the ninth month it is just below the xiphoid, and by the tenth month it has fallen back to its position in the eighth month.

The descent of the fetal head into the true pelvis, particularly in the primigravida, usually occurs about two weeks before term. This phenomenon, which suggests that the fetal head is not too large for the pelvis, is called *lightening*.

The uterus increases in *weight* from 60 g in the nonpregnant state to *1000* g at *term*. Myometrial fibers *stretch* and *hypertrophy* but undergo little if any hyperplasia. The myometrial fibers are disposed in *figure-of-eight* arrangements, which serve as living ligatures to effect hemostasis. Uterine *blood flow* increases to *600 ml/min* at term with a *parallel* increase in oxygen consumption. The *decidual reaction* involves hypertrophy of the endometrial glands and formation of large polygonal *stromal cells* filled with glycogen and lipid (decidual cells). Myometrial contractions progress from an irregular painless (Braxton Hicks) pattern to regular and painful contractions at term. The *basal cells* of the *cervical epithelium* undergo *hyperplasia*. The cervix increases in vascularity and softens as its glands hypertrophy. It remains occluded by a *mucous plug* until near the onset of labor. This mucus forms a beaded (cellular) rather than a fern pattern when allowed to dry on a glass slide.

A fern pattern is a manifestation of estrogenic dominance, which does not obtain in normal pregnancy. The estrogen is associated with a high content of electrolytes in the mucus, particularly sodium, which is responsible for the fern. As labor approaches, the cervix effaces and thins. In labor the external os dilates.

The growth of the uterus is a response to hormones in the first few months of pregnancy. Thereafter the growth is related to the mechanical effects of the enlarging products of conception. The uterus changes in shape from pyriform in the nonpregnant state to globular in early pregnancy and to ovoid in later pregnancy. It is frequently rotated laterally, more often to the right (dextrorotated).

The uterus increases in length from 7 cm in the nonpregnant state to 35 cm at term and from 500 to 1000 times in volume. The uteroplacental circulation develops as a low-resistance system. Uterine blood flow is only 1 to 2% of cardiac output in the nonpregnant state, whereas at the end of pregnancy it accounts for 20% of the cardiac output, which itself may be increased almost 50%. Uterine blood flow remains fairly constant, however, throughout the course of gestation when calculated in terms of flow to uterus and products of conception. The figure remains close to 10 to 15 ml/100 g of tissue/min. Oxygen consumption is fairly constant at 1 cc/100 g tissue/min.

The *vagina* undergoes an *increase* in *vascularity* early in pregnancy, developing a *bluish* discoloration that may aid in the diagnosis of pregnancy (p. 23). The increased production of *lactic acid* from glycogen by lactobacilli maintains the *acidic pH* of the vagina.

The primary change in the *ovary* is the formation of the *corpus luteum of pregnancy*, with accompanying *cessation of ovulation* and *menstruation*. The ovarian *vessels* undergo a huge *increase* in *caliber*.

The *breasts* undergo an increased *growth* of *ductal* and *alveolar* tissue. Development of the *ducts* is under the control of estrogen and that of the *alveoli* under the control of *progesterone*. Additional hormones involved in mammary development include prolactin, growth hormone, insulin, cortisone, and thyroxine. In addition to the general increase in size of breasts, areolae, and sebaceous glands (p. 22), the nipples enlarge and become more deeply pigmented and erectile.

The normal average *weight gain* in pregnancy is about *20 to 25 pounds*. Two pounds are normally gained in the first trimester and about 11 pounds in each of the last two trimesters. The average weight gain in pounds at term is distributed roughly as follows: fetus, 7.5; placenta, 1.0; amniotic fluid, 2.0; uterus, 2.5; breasts, 2.0; blood, 2.5; and interstitial fluid, 5.5.

The net gain in *protein* amounts to about *1 kg*, about half of which is in the products of conception and half in the uterus, breasts, and blood. About *seven liters* of *water* are retained until after delivery. Additional important metabolic changes include a *lowering of glucose tolerance* (p. 105), a *positive nitro-*

gen *balance*, and an *increase* in free fatty acids, phospholipids, and total *lipids*. The mother ordinarily needs about *800 mg of iron* during the course of gestation (500 mg for increased mass of maternal erythrocytes and 300 mg for the fetus and placenta).

Hypochlorhydria and vomiting in pregnancy may interfere with absorption of iron by the mother. The mother stores more calcium than the fetus requires until the last month of pregnancy, when the fetus needs about twice as much as the mother can ordinarily assimilate. The maternal reserves are then taxed and the mother may require additional calcium during lactation.

The *increase* in *blood volume* in pregnancy amounts to about *30* to *40%* above nonpregnant levels. The maximum is achieved at about *34 weeks* of gestation and is *maintained* throughout pregnancy without a terminal decrease. The elevation of the diaphragm with displacement of the heart to the left creates the false impression of cardiomegaly in normal pregnancy. *Increases* occur in *cardiac rate, stroke volume,* and *cardiac output.* The *circulation time* is somewhat *decreased.* Soft systolic apical and pulmonic *murmurs are common,* but *diastolic* murmurs indicate *disease* (p. 109).

The *rise* in *femoral venous pressure* is a result of *compression* of the *vena cava* by the enlarging uterus. *Arterial blood pressure*, however, is normally somewhat *decreased* in the *second trimester*.

The extent of the hemodynamic increases is as follows: erythrocyte mass, 25 to 30%; plasma volume, 40 to 50%; cardiac output, 30 to 40%; uterine blood flow, 1000%; and cardiac rate, 10 to 15 beats/min.

Hematocrit and *hemoglobin concentration* normally *decrease* as a result of the *hemodilution* of pregnancy. The *leukocyte count* may normally *increase* to 15,000 in pregnancy and to 25,000 in labor and the puerperium. There is no morphologic or numeric change in platelets, but *increases in fibrinogen*, and in Factors VII, VIII, IX, and X are found. An increased erythrocyte sedimentation rate and tendency to thrombosis may result from these changes.

Fibrinogen normally increases about 50% over nonpregnant levels from an average of 300 mg% to about 450 mg%. The decrease in concentration of plasma proteins amounts to about 1 g%. Most of the decrease is in the albumin fraction, with perhaps a slight increase in globulins. As a result, the A/G ratio falls. Among the numerous changes in serum enzymes, the increase in alkaline phosphatase is rather consistent.

Glomerular filtration rate (GFR) and *renal plasma flow* (RPF) both increase about 30 to 50% in normal pregnancy. Slight changes in glomerulotubular balance and in the load of filtered glucose result in frequent *glucosuria* in pregnancy. *Proteinuria*, however, is *abnormal.* Increased renal excretion results in *decrease* in *blood urea nitrogen* and *creatinine*. *Urinary stasis* results from *hypomotility* and dilatation of the ureters and renal pelves, a consequence primarily of the relaxation of smooth muscle by *progesterone*.

Dilatation of the ureter in pregnancy begins before the mechanical effect of the enlarging uterus is brought into play. The ureter in pregnancy is dilated, angulated, and elongated. The trigone of the bladder is elevated and edema of the base of the bladder predisposes to trauma. The combination of trauma and stasis leads to ascending infection of the urinary tract.

The increased GFR and progesterone tend to increase the excretion of sodium. Estrogen and corticosteroids tend to retain sodium. For accurate results in pregnancy the GFR and RPF must be measured in the lateral recumbent rather than the supine position.

Since *tidal volume* and *respiratory rate increase* in pregnancy, *minute volume* is *increased*. This *hyperventilation* may be a result of an increased sensitivity of the maternal respiratory center to carbon dioxide, perhaps as an effect of progesterone. *Respiratory alkalosis* may occur, but is *compensated* by a *decrease* in *serum bicarbonate* with resulting *stability* of *pH* of the blood.

Elevation of the diaphragm lowers the functional residual capacity, but vital capacity and maximum breathing capacity are not altered significantly.

Progesterone causes *decreased motility* of the *gastrointestinal tract* and *delayed absorption.*

Additional changes in the digestive tract include reduction in free HCl, reflux esophagitis, increased stasis in the gallbladder (possibly leading to formation of stones), and upward displacement of the appendix (possibly interfering with the diagnosis of acute appendicitis in pregnancy). Ptyalism (excessive salivation) and hyperemia of the gums, alterations in appetite, increased size of hemorrhoids, and constipation are commonly encountered in pregnancy.

General *endocrine changes* in pregnancy include *alterations* in *secretory* and *excretory rates,* in *binding* by *globulins,* and in *metabolic interactions,* and *increase* in *size* and *vascularity* of the endocrine organs. The most pronounced changes affect the *ovary,* with persistence of the corpus luteum, cessation of ovulation, and increased and prolonged elaboration of progesterone.

Moderate *enlargement* of the *thyroid gland* is accompanied by *increases in basal metabolic rate* (up to 25%), *protein-bound iodine* (50 to 100%), *butanol-extractable iodine, thyroid-binding globulin,* and *thyroxine. Triiodothyronine uptake* is *decreased* and *serum cholesterol increased. Free thyroxine* levels are essentially *unchanged.*

Pregnancy and hyperthyroidism share the following: increase in BMR, PBI, and RAI uptake; palpitation; tachycardia; perspiration; and emotional lability. Pregnancy and hyperthyroidism differ in the following respects: cholesterol is increased in pregnancy but decreased in hyperthyroidism; TBG is increased in pregnancy but is normal in hyperthyroidism; unbound thyroxine is not increased in pregnancy but is increased in hyperthyroidism; absolute iodine uptake is not increased in pregnancy but is increased in hyperthyroidism; and RBC-T_3 uptake is decreased in pregnancy but increased in hyperthyroidism.

The *pancreas* in pregnancy is subjected to a diabetogenic stress. Since islet cell function and *secretion* of *insulin* are *increased* while the *antagonism* of insulin by *placental lactogen* (*chorionic somatomammotropin*) *increases*, the pancreas is *taxed* in order to produce enough insulin to maintain the *hyperinsulinemia* of pregnancy (p. 105).

Production of *cortisol increases* although much of the steroid is *bound* by *transcortin*, which is increased in pregnancy. Some increase in free cortisol can be measured, however.

Aldosterone, renin substrate, renin (both concentration and activity), and angiotensin in plasma increase from twofold to tenfold. The increase in aldosterone protects against the natriuretic and antikaliuretic effects of progesterone. Enlargement of the adrenal cortex involves primarily the zona fasciculata, with the result that glucocorticoids but not 17-ketosteroids are considerably increased. The pituitary gland may enlarge sufficiently to compress the optic chiasma and reduce the visual fields. Parathormone levels are regulated by calcium levels in the blood, which ordinarily do not undergo great change.

Hyperpigmentation in pregnancy involves the areola, vulva, and linea nigra. Facial hyperpigmentation may result in *chloasma*, or the mask of pregnancy, which generally regresses post partum. These changes may be the result of an increase in melanocyte-stimulating hormone. *Striae* on the abdominal wall and breasts are *pink* during pregnancy, but may later become *silvery*, providing evidence of prior pregnancy. Vascular spiders and palmar erythema develop as effects of estrogen. Changes in the musculoskeletal system include progressive lumbar *lordosis*, with increased mobility of the pelvic joints and an anterior displacement of the center of gravity.

The commonly encountered increase in *emotional lability* is manifested by anxiety, apprehension, identity crises, and changes in libido. *Alterations* in *appetite* may include craving for unusual substances not normally considered as food (pica), such as starch and clay. *Postpartum depression* is common, although frank psychotic reactions reflect a preexisting tendency.

Gametogenesis and Fertilization

Somatic cells divide by *mitosis,* which results in two daughter cells with the same *diploid* number of chromosomes as the parent cell. *Gametogenesis* (*oogenesis* and *spermatogenesis*) requires *meiosis,* or reduction division, during which the chromosomal number is halved to produce *haploid* gametes. The *diploid* number is restored during *fertilization.*

Oogenesis begins in the fetus on the fifty-sixth day after conception, as oogonia enter prophase of the first meiotic division. The lengthy prophase in the female is divided into five phases: leptotene, zygotene, pachytene, diplotene, and diakinesis. During pachytene, the longest phase, pairing of homologous chromosomes and exchange of genetic material occur. At the end of the pachytene phase, oocytes enter the diplotene phase, in which they remain until they resume maturation or become atretic.

As many as seven million oocytes are present in the ovary during the fifth month of fetal development. At birth only two million remain. By the age of seven years the number is reduced to between 200,000 and 400,000. The decline continues throughout life, few oocytes surviving beyond menopause.

Primordial germ cells migrate from the endoderm of the yolk sac to the gonadal ridge, where they increase in number by mitotic division in the gonadal anlage. Oogonia are primordial germ cells that have ceased mitosis but have not yet entered the meiotic prophase. Upon entering prophase I, oogonia become primary oocytes, which when surrounded by a single layer of flattened follicular cells form primary follicles.

In each menstrual cycle between five and twenty follicles begin to develop but only one will ovulate. As many layers of follicular, or granulosa, cells are formed, spaces appear between the individual cells. As these spaces coalesce to form an antrum, the antral follicle develops. As the follicle enlarges and ovulation approaches, the mature, or graafian, follicle is formed. During folliculogenesis an acellular layer, the zona pellucida, is deposited around the oocyte by the granulosa cells.

During the follicular (proliferative) phase of the menstrual cycle, increasing titers of estradiol produced by the developing follicle eventually result in a surge of both FSH and LH from the pituitary. This release of pituitary hormones occurs on about day 14 of the normal cycle.

Follicle-stimulating hormone is a glycoprotein with a large sialic acid moiety and a half-life of about two hours. It is secreted by the basophilic cells of the anterior pituitary and is released by gonadotropin releasing hormone (GnRH). Negative feedback to estradiol occurs in both the pituitary and the hypothalamus. FSH effects follicular growth to the antral stage by promoting uptake of amino acids by the follicle. LH, probably through its steroidogenic action, is required for complete follicular maturation.

Luteinizing hormone is a glycoprotein with a small sialic acid moiety and a short half-life of about 30 minutes. It too is secreted by the basophilic cells of the anterior pituitary and released by the same gonadotropic releasing hormone that releases FSH. Negative feedback to progesterone and low levels of estradiol, and positive feedback to high levels of progesterone, as found in the mature graafian follicle, occur. The action of LH is to stimulate steroidogenesis in the ovary. High levels of LH, as in the preovulatory surge, inhibit formation of estrogen.

Follicular development depends on FSH, and the preovulatory surge of LH triggers resumption of meiotic activity within the oocyte. After the LH surge, the oocyte rapidly completes the first meiotic division, with production of a large secondary oocyte and a small first polar body. No synthesis of DNA occurs at this point and the secondary oocyte proceeds immediately to the metaphase of the second meiotic division, which is completed only after fertilization.

After ovulation the corpus luteum is formed. Inasmuch as release of the ovum from the follicle requires a greater concentration of LH than does formation of the corpus luteum, luteinization may sometimes occur without ovulation. Luteinization results in two changes in the ovary. The first is a change in the biosynthesis of steroids and the second is a proliferation of granulosa cells. In the follicular phase of the menstrual cycle, the follicle is capable of synthesizing estrogens from precursors of smaller molecular weight as well as from cholesterol. This pathway proceeds through the C_{21} steroids (which include progesterone) and the C_{19} compounds (which include testosterone) to C_{18} compounds (which include estradiol). In the luteal phase of the cycle, the granulosa cells lose the capacity to convert C_{21} compounds into C_{19} compounds. As a result of the change in biosynthetic pathways and the increased number of cells, a large amount of progesterone is released from the ovary. The theca interna, which secretes estrogen during the follicular phase, continues to produce estradiol during the luteal phase. The concentration of progesterone rises from the time of the midcycle surge of gonadotropin to a peak that occurs about seven days later. The variability in the length of the normal ovulatory cycle is a function primarily of the length of the follicular phase, for the corpus luteum has a finite life span of about 14 days. 

Development of spermatozoa begins with the spermatogonia, which comprise Type A and Type B elements. Spermatogonia of Type B divide mitotically to produce primary spermatocytes, which give rise through meiotic division to secondary spermatocytes and then haploid spermatids, half of which carry an X chromosome and half a Y. The process by which spermatids are transformed into spermatozoa is called spermiogenesis. When the spermatozoon achieves its definitive shape, it is released into the seminiferous tubule. Ability of the spermatozoon to fertilize is not achieved until its passage through the epididymis. The biochemical changes that render the spermatozoon capable of fertilization are known as capacitation, which occurs in the uterus, oviduct, or both. Capacitation is stimulated by estrogen and inhibited by progesterone.

Fertilization requires a capacitated spermatozoon, a mature secondary oocyte, and a milieu in which union of sperm and egg can occur. Fertilization generally occurs in the ampulla of the oviduct.

The secondary oocyte presents three barriers to spermatozoa: the mass of cumulus cells, the zona pellucida, and the vitelline membrane. In the process of penetration, spermatozoa must undergo the acrosome reaction. This reaction involves fusion of the plasma membrane of the spermatozoon with the outer acrosomal membrane, vesiculation of both membranes, and finally their disappearance. The result is the release of two enzymes: hyaluronidase, which disperses the cells of the cumulus and allows spermatozoa to reach the zona pellucida; and acrosin, a proteinase that lyses a path for the spermatozoon through the zona pellucida. After penetration by a spermatozoon, the Golgi apparatus of the oocyte disintegrates into small membrane-bound cortical granules, which migrate to a position immediately beneath the vitelline membrane. Release of material from the granules into the perivitelline space effects a block to polyspermy.

After fusion of the membranes of spermatozoon and ovum to form the *zygote*, meiosis resumes and the second polar body is extruded from the penetrated ovum. The haploid sets of chromosomes from spermatozoon and ovum are quickly surrounded by *pronuclear membranes* to form the male and female *pronuclei*. Fertilization is completed when the pronuclei move to the center of the zygote, the pronuclear membranes disintegrate, and the maternal and paternal chromosomes are aligned on the metaphase plate of the first cleavage division. In the human being, the *two-cell* stage is not attained until *24 to 36* hours after fertilization.

The ovulated oocyte normally remains capable of being fertilized for not longer than 12 hours. Although it may be penetrated at a later stage, it will probably degenerate before implantation. Breakdown of the metaphase II spindle may result in trisomy or failure of extrusion of the second polar body (triploidy). During aging of the oocyte, cortical granules move toward the center of the oocyte, where they are no longer in a position to block polyspermy.

Early Development of the Fetus

For the first 24 hours after fertilization the zygote remains in the *one-cell* stage. The *two-cell* stage begins 24 hours after fertilization and ends 12 hours later. The *four-cell* stage lasts from hour 36 to hour 48; the *eight-cell* stage lasts from hour 48 to hour 72; and the *16-cell* stage lasts from hour 72 to hour 96. The zygote enters the uterine cavity as a solid ball of cells, the *morula*, between three and five days after fertilization. In the uterus the morula is transformed into a fluid-filled *blastocyst*, which consists of an outer covering of *trophoblast* and a small *inner cell mass* (embryo-forming cells). The *zona pellucida* is lost at this stage and the blastocyst then implants on around day 6 with the *embryonic pole* in contact with the endometrium. During the second week the *bilaminar embryo* is formed and during the third week the *trilaminar embryo* develops. The *embryonic period* comprises the second through the eighth weeks and the *fetal period* the remainder of gestation (third through tenth lunar months).

By day 16 the trilaminar embryonic disc comprises ectoderm, endoderm, and mesoderm. At about day 20 the paraxial mesoderm begins to divide into paired cuboidal bodies called somites, the primordia of the axial skeleton and associated musculature. Each column of paraxial mesoderm is continuous laterally with the intermediate mesoderm, the primordia of the urogenital system (p. 199). Laterally, the intermediate mesoderm thins and becomes continuous with the lateral mesoderm, the primordia of the body wall and the wall of the primitive gut.

The most significant event in the establishment of general form of the developing body occurs during the embryonic period, namely, the process of folding, which transforms the flat, oblong trilaminar disc into a cylindrical embryo. This folding in both longitudinal and transverse planes is caused by rapid growth in the region of the neural tube, a slower rate of growth at the periphery of the embryonic disc, and a slight constriction in the region of the future umbilical cord.

Development of the Placenta and Fetal Membranes

The human placenta is basically a *chorioallantoic* structure, for although a vesicular allantois is lacking, the precociously developed allantoic mesenchyme, which later forms the *um-*

bilical cord, gives rise in situ to the allantoic vessels that vascularize the chorion. Because maternal blood is in direct contact with trophoblast-covered villi, the human placenta is classified as *hemochorial.*

The yolk sac, or umbilical vesicle into which it develops, is prominent at the beginning of pregnancy. The embryo is at first a flattened disc, situated between amnion and yolk sac. As the embryo grows, it bulges into the amnionic sac, and the dorsal part of the yolk sac is incorporated into the body of the embryo to form the gut. The yolk sac may occasionally be recognized even in the mature placenta as a crumpled vascular sac between amnion and chorion.

The allantois may project into the base of the body stalk. Its mesoderm normally contains two arteries and one vein. The right umbilical vein disappears early, leaving only the original left vein.

The amnion forms around the eighth day of development by cavitation. Distention of its sac brings the amnion into contact with the internal surface of the chorion. Apposition of the mesoblasts of chorion and amnion occurs between the fourth and fifth months of gestation with the result that the extraembryonic celom is obliterated.

The changes that culminate in the transformation of the endometrium to *decidua* are not complete until several days after *implantation* (nidation). Directly beneath the site of implantation is the *decidua basalis.* Surrounding the ovum and separating it from the rest of the uterine cavity, in the early months of gestation, is the *decidua capsularis,* which forms as a result of *deep,* or *interstitial,* implantation. The remainder of the pregnant uterus is lined by *decidua parietalis.*

The human blastocyst is completely embedded in the endometrium by day 11 or 12. The greater part of the chorion, in contact with the decidua capsularis, loses its villi between the third and fourth months of gestation and forms the smooth chorion, or *chorion laeve.* The villi on the side of the chorion toward the decidua basalis enlarge and become elaborately branched to form the *chorion frondosum.* By the third month the decidua capsularis degenerates and the chorion laeve comes into contact with the parietal decidua of the opposite wall of the uterus. The human placenta is thus of *dual origin*, comprising fetal (chorion frondosum) and maternal (decidua basalis) elements.

Once the cytotrophoblast has penetrated the deepest layer of decidua, continued growth of normal placenta cannot be accomplished by further trophoblastic invasion. Increased thickness of the placenta must therefore be the result of growth in length and size of the villi of the chorion frondosum, with accompanying expansion of the intervillous space. Until the end of the fourth month, the placenta grows in thickness and circumference; thereafter, there is no appreciable increase in thickness, but growth in circumference continues almost throughout pregnancy.

The earliest form of nutrition is derived from *endometrial secretion;* later, *maternal blood* is the source. During and after implantation there appear within the *syncytiotrophoblast* numerous vacuoles, the coalescence of which creates *lacunae*, which merge to form the *intervillous space*. Maternal venous sinuses are tapped early, but until day 14 or 15 no arterial blood enters the intervillous space. By day 17 the chorionic villi are *vascularized*, but until villous and fetal vessels are connected and the fetal cardiac pulsations are initiated (in the second month), no true *circulation* can be described.

Villi may first be distinguished on or about day 12. The period between days 9 and 20 is characterized by intense growth and differentiation of the chorion. The trophoblastic trabeculae develop a cellular core as a result of multiplication of *cytotrophoblastic elements*. These highly modified trabeculae may then be designated *primary villi*. The villous stems later develop mesodermal cores, which convert primary into *secondary* villi. Vascularization of the secondary villi transforms them into *tertiary* villi, the principal organs of exchange in the human placenta. Proliferation of cellular trophoblast at the tips of the villi forms the cytotrophoblastic *cell columns*, which are not invaded by mesenchyme but are anchored to the decidua at the *basal plate*.

Fetoplacental Physiology

The fetus derives all its *nutrition* from the mother through the *placenta,* which serves as a fetal kidney, liver, lung, and endocrine organ. The unusual *dual circulation* of the placenta allows for effective fetomaternal exchange. Maternal blood enters the basal plate of the placenta, whence it is driven by the maternal systolic blood pressure toward the *chorionic plate.* As the blood falls back toward the basal plate, exchange takes place. The deoxygenated blood then returns to the uterine veins through the *basal plate.*

The unique features of the placenta include its *extracorporeal* location, its *limited life span,* its *multiplicity* of *functions,* and its apparent *immunologic hyporeactivity.* The retention of fetal (placental) tissue within the mother for a period of time far exceeding that of homograft rejection depends primarily on the special properties of the *trophoblast.* An absence or a deficiency of trophoblastic histocompatibility antigens, presence of extracellular sialomucin coatings of the trophoblast, and perhaps effects of progesterone and immunologic enhancement are principal factors in retention of the foreign tissue.

The trophoblast produces both *protein* and *steroid* hormones. The proteins are synthesized by the trophoblastic *syncytium;* synthesis of the steroids involves participation by the *mother* and *fetus* as well as the syncytium. The level of *human chorionic gonadotropin* (hCG) is elevated abruptly in early pregnancy, reaching a *peak* at about *80 days* and gradually declining to a level that remains low throughout pregnancy. The production of hCG by the trophoblast is the basis for hormonal pregnancy tests (p. 23).

Chorionic gonadotropin is a glycoprotein with a large sialic acid moiety, which gives it a long half-life of 6 to 24 hours. This hormone has primarily LH-like properties on bioassay, with lesser FSH-like activity. It substitutes for pituitary gonadotropins in maintaining steroidogenesis in the corpus luteum of pregnancy.

Chorionic gonadotropin reaches a peak of 100,000 to 300,000 IU/liter of maternal urine by the end of the second month of pregnancy. By the fourth month the level is down to

25,000 to 50,000 IU/liter. A low level is maintained to term. Between 45 minutes and six days after expulsion of the placenta, hCG normally disappears from the urine.

The other important protein hormone is *human placental lactogen* (hPL), also named *human chorionic somatomammotropin* (hCS), which undergoes a *gradual increase* from six weeks' gestation to term. It is *diabetogenic* and bears a physiologic and chemical resemblance to human growth hormone.

Placental lactogen is a polypeptide with both prolactin-like and growth-hormone-like activities. It may substitute for prolactin in supporting ovarian function in early pregnancy and may promote development of the breast, inasmuch as growth hormone is necessary for expression of the effects of estrogen and progesterone on mammary tissue.

The plasma level of hPL reaches a maximum of between 20 and 25 μg/ml near term. The level of this hormone may be an index of placental function. Levels below 4 μg/ml after the thirtieth week of gestation have been associated in some but not all studies with poor perinatal outcome.

Progesterone is synthesized by the placenta from *maternal precursors*. This steroid, which is essential for the maintenance of pregnancy, gradually increases to term. The main *estrogen* excreted in pregnancy is *estriol*. Its production requires a supply of *androgens* by the fetal *adrenal cortex* and metabolic participation by the *fetal liver* and *placenta*. Its level rises throughout pregnancy with a sharp *increase at 28 weeks*. Defective function of the fetal adrenal or liver or of the placenta may lead to low levels of estriol in the maternal urine or plasma.

The principal metabolite of progesterone in pregnancy is pregnanediol, which reaches a maximum at about 32 weeks' gestation. It is not a reliable index of placental function. At the fourteenth week of pregnancy the maternal excretion of urinary estrogen is 1 mg/day. At term the level is normally 30 mg/day, about 90% of which is estriol (E_3).

Maternal cholesterol is converted to pregnenolone by the placenta. This compound is then converted to dehydroisoandrosterone sulfate (DHAS) by the fetal adrenal. DHAS is then hydroxylated at the 16-position in the fetal liver. This is the rate-limiting reaction. The 16-alpha-OH-DHA is converted to estriol in the placenta. It is conjugated to a glucosiduronate or a sulfate and is excreted as E_3G in the maternal urine. The placenta does not synthesize corticosteroids. A TSH-like activity in the placenta may be one of the numerous effects of chorionic gonadotropin. The placenta is somewhat permeable to thyroxine but not to TSH, parathormone, posterior pituitary extract, or insulin.

Placental *transfer* in either direction may be *active* or *passive.* The rate of transfer depends principally on the following factors: the *rates* of *maternal* and *fetal blood flows,* the respective *concentrations* of substances in the *maternal* and *fetal plasmas* (concentration gradients), the *area* and *thickness* of the placental *membrane,* the *molecular weight* and *electrical* charge of the compound, the *physical properties* of the barrier, the *biochemical mechanisms* for active transfer, and the *metabolism* by the *placenta* itself.

Since most *drugs* administered to the mother, including *antibiotics* and *anesthetics,* as well as *gases, nutrients,* many *hormones,* and *some immunoglobulins,* cross the placenta, everything prescribed for the mother during pregnancy must be considered in terms of effects on the fetus as well. A few agents, such as *succinylcholine, d-tubocurarine,* and *heparin,* however, cross *very slightly* or not at all. Other substances are concentrated preferentially in the fetal circulation.

The fetus meets its requirements for *iron* even in the presence of maternal anemia. It maintains *oxygenation* of its blood by several mechanisms. First, fetal erythrocytes have a *higher affinity for oxygen* than do maternal erythrocytes. The *higher hemoglobin level* of the newborn resembles that seen in the adult at high altitude. Fetal blood has a *greater oxygen capacity,* but has a *lower saturation* and a *higher hematocrit* than does adult blood. Accumulation of iron in the fetal liver occurs mainly in the third trimester.

Placental transfer occurs as a result of several mechanisms. Respiratory gases and some electrolytes are transferred by simple diffusion. Sodium is probably transferred actively, with chloride then diffusing to maintain electrostatic balance. Carbohydrates are transferred by facilitated diffusion, and amino acids and some vitamins by active transport. Ascorbic acid, for example, is concentrated on the fetal side. Differential rates of transfer of stereoisomers, such as D- and L-histidine, are evidence of enzyme-mediated carrier mechanisms. In general, the greater the degree of lipid solubility and the smaller the molecular weight, the greater is the rate of transfer. Certain molecules of high molecular weight, however, such as some of the immunoglobulins, cross the placenta, whereas others of equal molecular weight do not. In general, uncharged particles are transferred more readily. Macromolecules may be transported across the placenta by pinocytosis. Water is transferred by bulk flow in response to small hydrostatic or osmotic pressure gradients. Breaks in placental villi lead to leakage of fetal erythrocytes into the maternal circulation and possible Rh-isoimmunization in certain circumstances (p. 103). Some viruses such as rubella may cross the placenta and produce fetal disease (p. 111).

IgG passes the placenta, whereas IgM and IgA do not. Passive immunity to some diseases may be conferred on the fetus as a result of the transfer of these antibodies. In addition, the fetus may produce some of its own antibodies after midpregnancy.

The fetus receives most of its nitrogen as amino acids and synthesizes its own protein. Although the placenta transfers phospholipids, which are subsequently degraded, most of the fetal lipid is synthesized by the fetus itself. Similarly, the fetus synthesizes its own nucleic acids. Glucose is readily transferred in both directions, but the maternal level is usually higher than the fetal. The levels of calcium and phosphorus, however, are higher on the fetal side.

A fetus reaches *term* at *40 weeks*. It is considered *mature* at *2500 g*, which corresponds to about *36 weeks'* gestation. It is sometimes considered *viable* at *500 g*, which corresponds to about midpregnancy.

The fetal hypogastric arteries continue extraabdominally as umbilical arteries, which carry deoxygenated blood to the placenta. The umbilical vein carries relatively well-oxygenated blood from the placenta back to the fetus. Various shunts of oxygenated blood characterize the fetal circulation. Some blood from the umbilical vein is shunted through the ductus venosus to avoid the liver, the only organ to receive undiluted freshly oxygenated blood. The upper half of the fetal body receives more oxygen than does the lower half. The foramen ovale shunts blood to the left side of the heart to supply the head. The ductus arteriosus shunts much of the pulmonary arterial flow to the aorta, thus bypassing the lungs.

At birth, the lungs expand as the infant draws its first breath. As blood begins to flow through the pulmonary vessels, the ductus venosus, foramen ovale, and ductus arteriosus undergo functional closure.

The high cardiac output of the fetus and the high hemoglobin content and better oxygen dissociation of fetal hemoglobin compensate for the relatively poor oxygen content of fetal blood. The fetal heart rate of 135/min drops to about 110/min in the newborn.

By the third month of fetal life, the genitalia are sufficiently differentiated to allow diagnosis of sex. By the second trimester the liver has replaced the placenta as the principal organ for storage of carbohydrate.

The growth of the fetus by weight and length is as follows:

Gestational Week	Length (cm) (Crown-heel)	Weight (g)
8	3	1
12	10	18
16	18	100
20	25	300
24	32	600
28	37	1000
32	42	1700
36	47	2500
40	50	3200 or more

The composition of the *amniotic fluid* is determined in part by metabolic products of the fetus. The fluid is *at first isotonic* with maternal serum and is *later* diluted by *hypotonic* fetal urine. The volume of fluid increases to a maximum of slightly over 1000 ml at about 35 weeks and gradually decreases to between 500 and 800 ml at term. Examination of the amniotic fluid can be used to assess *fetal well-being* and *maturity*. The *cells* and *fluid* are examined to detect sex of the fetus and many metabolic and *chromosomal* abnormalities.

Fetal maturity may be assessed by a variety of clinical and laboratory methods. An accurate knowledge of the LMP and time of onset of quickening, inspection and palpation of the maternal abdomen to assess size, and radiologic demonstration of bony epiphyses are helpful. One of the most accurate techniques, with an error of only 2 mm, is measurement of the fetal biparietal diameter by ultrasound. A diameter of 9.0 cm or more usually indicates a mature fetus weighing 2500 g or more. Circumferences of the head, chest, and abdomen may also be measured sonographically. Several chemical studies of the amniotic fluid have proved fairly reliable in ascertaining fetal age. The concentration of creatinine should be 2 mg% or more after the thirty-seventh week of gestation. In the normal term fetus the bilirubin concentration should be negligible. In the mature fetus the osmolality, which is measured by depression of the freezing point and reflects predominantly the concentration of sodium, should be less than 250 milliosmoles. The lecithin/sphingomyelin ratio is approximately 1.0 at the thirty-fifth week. An L/S ratio of about 2.0 indicates pulmonary maturity and little likelihood of respiratory distress syndrome. A lower ratio, however, does not necessarily indicate the likely development of respiratory distress syndrome. Measurements of the L/S ratio are of limited value in diabetic pregnancies. In such cases it is of greater prognostic significance to measure specifically the level of dipalmitoyl lecithin. A "shake test" to detect bubbles in the amniotic fluid may be employed as a rough guide to the presence of surface-active substances. The number of cells stained orange with Nile blue sulfate provides a crude estimate of fetal maturity.

Examination of the amniotic fluid and cells can be used for

the following additional purposes: detection of biochemical disorders (enzymatic defects) such as Tay-Sachs disease; ascertaining fetal blood type; detection of the sex of the fetus (by Barr body analysis or karyotype) in cases of sex-linked disorders; and detection of chromosomal disorders (by karyotype analysis), such as Down's syndrome in fetuses of elderly mothers.

In a description of the karyotype the first item to be recorded is the total number of chromosomes (including sex chromosomes) followed by a comma (,). The sex chromosomal constitution is recorded after the comma:

46,XX	Normal female
46,XY	Normal male
45,X	Turner's syndrome
47,XXY	Klinefelter's syndrome

Numerical aberrations of the autosomes are indicated by the group letter or individual chromosomal number followed by a plus (+) or minus (−) sign after the sex chromosomal designation:

45,XX,C−	45 chromosomes, XX sex chromosomes, a missing C-group chromosome
46,XY,18+21−	46 chromosomes, XY sex chromosomes, an extra chromosome 18 and a missing chromosome 21

Chromosomal mosaicism is indicated by two karyotypic designations separated by a diagonal (/):

45,X/46,XY	A chromosomal mosaic with two cell types—one with 45 chromosomes and a single X and the other with 46 chromosomes and XY sex chromosomes
46,XY/47,XY,G+	A chromosomal mosaic with a normal male cell line and a cell line with an extra G-group chromosome

The short arm of a chromosome is designated by the lowercase letter "p" and the long arm by the letter "q." Increase in the length of an arm of a chromosome is indicated by placing a plus (+) sign and decrease in length by placing a minus (−) sign after the designation of the arm:

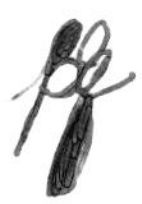

46,XX,2p+	46 chromosomes with an increase in length of the short arm of chromosome 2

A translocation is indicated by the letter "t" followed by parentheses, which include the chromosomes involved:

46,XY,t(Bp−;Dq+) or 46,XX,t(Bp+;Dq−)	A balanced reciprocal translocation between the short arm of a B-group chromosome and the long arm of a D-group chromosome

In a centric fusion translocation in which only one translocation chromosome is present, the semicolon is omitted:

45,XX,D−,G−,t(DqGq)+	45 chromosomes, XX sex chromosomes, one chromosome missing from the D-group and one from the G-group, their long arms having united to form a DG translocation chromosome

Trisomy 21 (47,XX,+21, or 47, XY,+21) is the most common trisomy compatible with life. It accounts for 95% of all cases of Down's syndrome and is found in one in about 800 births. Virtually all affected persons are mentally retarded and 30% have congenital cardiac disease. Less common forms of Down's syndrome involve translocations and mosaicism.

Several classes of inherited biochemical disorders are detectable in the middle trimester through analysis of fluid obtained by amniocentesis. Among the disorders of lipid metabolism are Gaucher's disease, GM_2 gangliosidosis type I (Tay-Sachs disease), and the varieties of Niemann-Pick's disease. The disorders of carbohydrate metabolism include galactosemia, glucose-6-phosphate dehydrogenase deficiency, and the glycogen storage diseases. Disorders resulting from disturbances in mucopolysaccharide metabolism are Hurler's, Hunter's, Sanfilippo's, and Morquio's syndromes. Inborn errors of amino acid and organic acid metabolism include homocystinuria, maple syrup urine disease, methylmalonic acidemia, and phenylketonuria. The Lesch-Nyhan syndrome is listed among the miscellaneous disorders.

Dysmaturity is a discrepancy between birth weight and gestational age. It is associated with increased perinatal mortality and morbidity. The obstetrician must identify predisposing factors and the pediatrician must treat the often associated hypoglycemia and acidosis and detect anomalies. The dysmature infant has peeling skin, loss of subcutaneous tissue, and dystrophic nails.

Many maternal, placental, and fetal factors are associated with intrauterine growth retardation. The more important include the following: hypoperfusion of the placenta; maternal undernutrition and hypoxia; low maternal socioeconomic status; small size of the mother; maternal smoking during pregnancy; high altitude; maternal disorders, including cardiac disease, pulmonary insufficiency, essential hypertension, preeclampsia, chronic renal disease, some hemoglobinopathies, thyrotoxicosis, and phenylketonuria; transplacental viral infection, for example rubella or cytomegalovirus; chromosomal abnormalities in the fetus, including trisomies and deletion syndromes; and prolonged pregnancy.

Antepartum Care

A major purpose of antepartum care is *education* of the patient about *pregnancy, labor,* and *delivery.* Pregnancy should be explained as a *physiologic process* rather than an illness. The antepartum period is a good time to practice *preventive medicine,* since ideally the patient is under a physician's supervision for at least half a year. During this time *dental care* may be obtained, an adequate *diet* planned, and advice about *sexual activity* and *contraception* given.

An exemplary diet should be planned in detail to ensure a *well-balanced menu* including meat, eggs, fresh fruits and vegetables, and a total intake of 2500 calories. Iron should be prescribed with meals (p. 114). Prenatal vitamins may be given routinely, although a well-balanced diet with iron supplementation is usually adequate for a healthy woman.

The patient should be told that *bathing* is permissible, especially since bath water does not enter the vagina, and that coitus may be continued, if desired, so long as there are no abnormalities of pregnancy and it causes no discomfort. *Normal physical activity* should be permitted to the point of fatigue. The patient should be encouraged to *walk* about a half mile a day and to continue work as long as she is physically and emotionally comfortable. *Short-distance travel* may be permitted, but long trips should be undertaken only with the doctor's knowledge and consent.

Classes for both parents are valuable to allay fear of labor and delivery. The patient should be informed that any *drug* taken during pregnancy may *affect the fetus* (Table 4). The obstetrician must therefore be consulted before the patient undergoes any diagnostic investigation or treatment. She should receive *no immunizations* with *live virus* during pregnancy. Vaccines with killed organisms and tetanus *toxoid* may be administered during pregnancy.

During the antepartum course the various methods of analgesia and anesthesia should be discussed and the patient informed about the available forms of contraception. She should be given the opportunity to decide whether she prefers *breast feeding* the baby or a bottle. She should also be encouraged to select possible *names* for the baby. The patient must be taught to recognize the *onset of labor,* that is, the regular, painful, progressive contractions, and to report any *"bloody show"* (blood-tinged mucous discharge from the vagina that accompanies dilatation of the cervix during the first stage of labor) or rupture of the membranes (definite or suspected). The patient should be instructed to take *no food* after the onset of labor. It is important that the patient be taught to report any of the *danger signs* of pregnancy, including *vaginal bleeding, abdominal pain, edema, blurred vision, headache,* or any significant *change in well-being.*

An exemplary daily diet should contain about 150 g of carbohydrate, 100 g of fat, and 85 g of protein. Six to eight glasses of

TABLE 4. Effects of Maternal Drugs and Diseases on the Fetus and Newborn

MATERNAL DRUG OR DISEASE	EFFECT
Alcohol	Growth deficiencies; mental retardation
Amethopterin	Anomalies; abortion
Ammonium chloride	Acidosis
Androgens	Masculinization
Cephalothin	Positive direct Coombs' test
Chlorambucil	Anomalies; abortion
Chloramphenicol	"Gray baby syndrome"
Coumadin	Fetal death; hemorrhage
Cytomegalic inclusion disease	Fetal death; mental retardation
Diuretics	Electrolyte imbalance
Heroin	Neonatal death or convulsions
Hexamethonium	Neonatal ileus
Methimazole	Goiter; mental retardation
Morphine	Neonatal death or convulsions
Novobiocin	Hyperbilirubinemia
Phenobarbital	Neonatal bleeding
Potassium iodide	Goiter; mental retardation
Progestins	Masculinization
Propylthiouracil	Goiter; mental retardation
Reserpine	Nasal congestion and drowsiness
Rubella	Cardiac, ocular, and otologic abnormalities; mental retardation
Salicylates (excess)	Neonatal bleeding
Smallpox vaccination	Fetal vaccinia
Smoking	Light babies (low weight)
Streptomycin	Acoustic nerve damage
Sulfonamides	Kernicterus
Syphilis	Rhinorrhea; conjunctivitis; congenital syphilis
Tetracyclines	Discoloration of teeth; inhibition of bone growth
Thalidomide	Phocomelia
Thiazides	Thrombocytopenia
Toxoplasmosis	Chorioretinitis; hydrocephalus; CNS calcification
Varicella-zoster	Intrauterine and persistent postnatal disease
Vitamin K analogues (excess)	Hyperbilirubinemia

fluid and a quart of milk a day are desirable. The diet should specifically contain adequate amounts of calcium, iron, vitamin A, thiamine, riboflavin, niacin, folic acid, and vitamins C and D. The sodium content of carbonated beverages and beer and the caloric content of alcohol must be considered in planning the diet. Consumption of alcohol should be limited to two ounces of whiskey, or the equivalent of other alcoholic beverages, per day. If specific dietary problems arise, a professional dietician should be consulted.

A maternity girdle and low-heeled walking shoes may add to the patient's comfort. No hand-bulb syringes must be used for douching because of the danger of air embolism, and the douche bag should be held not more than two feet above the level of the hips to avoid undue pressure. Coitus may be continued unless premature labor, rupture of the membranes, vaginal bleeding, or infection supervenes. Cunnilingus during pregnancy may introduce air into the vagina and cause fatal air embolism.

An important aspect of antepartum care is *identification* of the *high-risk* pregnancy. First, a *history* of medical, surgical, or obstetric complications in prior pregnancies must be elicited. Risk is increased in patients of *low socioeconomic status* and possibly unwed mothers, in whom the effects of environment and heredity are often difficult to separate. *Extremes of age* (under 15 and over 40) are associated with more obstetric complications. *Obesity*, addiction or habituation to *drugs*, and heavy intake of *ethanol* are all associated with an increased rate of complications. *Heavy smoking* by the mother leads to *lighter* but not necessarily premature *infants*. *High parity itself*, moreover, is associated with a significantly increased rate of obstetric complications.

In obtaining the obstetric history the doctor should inquire specifically about diabetes mellitus, tuberculosis, rheumatic fever, cardiac disease, renal disease, syphilis, rubella, pelvic operations, hereditary diseases, and a familial history of twins. History of the menses and prior pregnancies should be recorded in detail.

Many findings obtained on *examination* of the *mother* give clues to high-risk pregnancy. The more important include:

abnormal growth of the uterus (suggesting plural gestation, hydramnios, and hydatidiform mole), dead fetus, contracted pelvis, abnormal presentation, and large or abnormal fetuses. *Fetal indications* of a high-risk pregnancy include retardation of growth and abnormal heart sounds.

Laboratory tests used to detect possible complications of pregnancy include: serologic test for syphilis, examination of urine for glucose and protein, urine culture (particularly with a history of urologic infection), hemoglobin and hematocrit, Papanicolaou smear, glucose tolerance test in the presence of glycosuria or a history suggestive of diabetes, and culture for gonorrhea obtained from urethra, cervix, and anus. Fetal disease may be anticipated by identifying the mother's blood group (ABO) and Rh-type. In cases of Rh-negative mothers, antibody titers are indicated (p. 103).

Antepartum visits should be made monthly during the first six months, every two weeks from the twenty-eighth to the thirty-sixth week of gestation, and weekly during the last month. The patient should *consult* the *obstetrician* as *early* in pregnancy as possible. The advantages include early accurate diagnosis of the onset of pregnancy and careful surveillance during the period of early fetal growth. In the first few months of pregnancy the fetus is most susceptible to the effects of ingested drugs and environmental factors such as irradiation.

Accurate records must be kept in an effort to optimize maternal and fetal well-being. The patient must be encouraged to *ask questions* during her visits and the obstetrician must answer them factually and completely. Several suitable books are readily available to provide further information to the patient.

At each antepartum visit the *blood pressure, weight,* and *urinary protein* should be checked, primarily to detect *preeclampsia* (p. 99). The normal midtrimester drop in blood pressure should be recognized. Weight gain is normally kept to *20 to 25 pounds,* but in the absence of fluid retention a greater weight gain in itself may not be harmful to the outcome of the pregnancy. In no case should the patient be placed on a program of weight reduction, and "diet pills" of all varieties are contraindicated in pregnancy. In cases of suspected recent exposure to *rubella, antibody titers* should be obtained (p. 111).

At later visits the *height of the fundus* should be carefully noted and the *fetal heart tones recorded* (by stethoscope or

Doptone). The presence of plural gestation or abnormalities of presentation should be noted as soon as they are suspected. In the third trimester it is appropriate to *repeat* the *hemoglobin*, the serologic test for *syphilis*, and the *gonococcal* cultures. The *chest film* should be deferred normally until after the fifth month to minimize the risk of radiation to the fetus. A *pelvic examination* including *Papanicolaou smear* is performed at the initial visit, but it may be easier to perform *manual pelvimetry* later in pregnancy when the pelvic tissues are more relaxed. If small measurements are detected clinically, roentgenologic pelvimetry may be indicated.

Manual pelvimetry should include an estimate of the diagonal conjugate (the distance from the promontory of the sacrum to the inferior border of the pubic symphysis), which is normally about 12.5 cm. The true conjugate is the distance from the promontory of the sacrum to the superior border of the symphysis. It cannot be measured manually, but is estimated by subtracting between 1 and 2 cm from the diagonal conjugate, depending on the height and inclination of the symphysis, to give a figure of about 11 cm. The intertuberous diameter (the distance between the inner aspects of the ischial tuberosities) is the transverse diameter of the outlet and is generally about 11 cm. If the diagonal conjugate is below 11.5 cm, further study is often indicated (p. 95).

Other pelvic features of obstetric importance are the shape of the pubic arch, the width of the sacrosciatic notch, the prominence of the ischial spines, the shape of the forepelvis, the convergence of the side walls, and the thickness of the bones. X-ray pelvimetry may be indicated for small or abnormal pelves, a floating fetal head at term in a primigravida, a history of difficult forceps deliveries, and a primigravida with a breech presentation.

In discussing common complaints with the patient it is important to distinguish *physiologic alterations* of pregnancy from *disease* and to *discourage* the use of *drugs* whenever possible. Lassitude, urinary frequency without dysuria, ptyalism, tingling of the breasts, palpitation, tachypnea, and occasional syncope ordinarily require *no special therapy*. Backache may be relieved by supportive garments and a firm mattress. *Constipation* may be treated with mild laxatives, a high intake of fluids, and a diet high in bulk. *Varicosities* may require supportive stockings and elevation of the legs. Leukorrhea, hemorrhoids, and heartburn occasionally require symptomatic therapy. Painful uterine contractions must be distinguished by continued observation from true progressive labor (p. 90). Any *severe abdominal pain*, however, requires ruling out appendicitis, cholecystitis, partial abruption of the placenta, and urinary tract infection.

Pica, which may interfere with a regular diet, should be recognized and discouraged. *Emotional liability*, as opposed to a true psychiatric disturbance, usually responds well to simple support and reassurance.

Hyperemesis gravidarum is an exaggeration of nausea and vomiting of pregnancy, with systemic effects such as acetonuria and substantial weight loss. It is best treated with multiple small feedings high in carbohydrates and sometimes antiemetics.

Hyperemesis gravidarum appears to be less common than formerly and is no longer considered a form of preeclampsia. Etiologic factors may include elevated levels of gonadotropins and steroids, delayed gastric emptying, and emotional predisposition. It is most common between the second and fourth months of pregnancy. The important components of therapy include maintenance of fluid and electrolyte balance, correction of other diseases, and avoidance of obnoxious odors. Other causes of nausea and vomiting must be ruled out, including viral hepatitis and ulcers. Hyperemesis gravidarum is often associated with immature personalities but is not apparently increased in unwed mothers. Psychologic support is important and antiemetic agents such as cyclizine, meclizine, and dicyclomine may be useful and have not proved to be teratogenic. Drastic and punitive measures have no place in the management of hyperemesis, and abortion is rarely indicated.

Labor and Delivery

Labor is divided into *three stages*. The *first stage* begins with the onset of true labor and ends with *full dilatation* of the cervix (10 cm). The *second stage* begins with full dilatation of the cervix and ends with *birth* of the *fetus.* The *third stage* begins with birth of the fetus and ends with the *expulsion* or *extraction* of the *placenta* and *membranes.*

Labor is characterized by *progressive dilatation* and effacement of the cervix, which accompany *regular* painful uterine *contractions* normally associated with *descent* of the *presenting part* (that part of the fetus that is lowest in the pelvis). The presenting part is the part of the fetus that is palpated by the examining finger on vaginal or rectal examination, for example, occiput, sacrum, or acromion. *Dilatation* of the cervix is the enlargement of the *external* cervical *os* caused by the upward *retraction* of the *myometrial fibers* during labor. *Effacement* of the cervix is accomplished when the cervix is completely retracted, the cervicovaginal angle has disappeared, and only the external os remains to be dilated.

Labor is divided into *active* and *latent* phases. The latent phase is the time between the onset of regular uterine contractions and appreciable cervical dilatation. During this phase the cervix effaces but dilates only slightly. The active phase extends from the end of the latent phase to the end of the first stage of labor. The events of labor normally occur in an *orderly* sequence at *accelerating* rates. Variations from this pattern may indicate impending abnormalities (p. 90).

Normal uterine contractions are characterized by *fundal dominance* (contractions that are strongest in the top of the uterus and weakest in the bottom) and *symmetry* (contractions that arise simultaneously from both cornual areas). The *intensity* of normal uterine contractions increases progressively so that at the height of a contraction the myometrium can be indented only with strong digital pressure. The *tonus* of the uterus is the pressure between contractions, when the myometrium can be indented with only moderate digital pressure. The *frequency* of uterine contractions gradually increases to about one every two to three minutes and the *duration* to between 45 and 60 seconds at the end of labor.

The *upper segment* of the uterus is the *thick contractile* portion; the *lower segment* is *thin* and *passive.* A *retraction ring* may divide the two.

The first stage of labor is concerned with overcoming cervical resistance and the second stage with the passage of the fetus through the birth canal. Although the lengths of the stages of labor may normally vary within fairly wide limits, the first stage lasts about six to eight hours in the multipara and 10 to 14 hours in the primigravida. The second stage should not last longer than two hours. The third stage usually lasts about 15 to 30 minutes and should be terminated after one hour at the latest.

The three main factors determining the course of labor are the *powers* (uterine contractions), the *passages* (bony pelvis and maternal soft tissues), and the *passenger* (size and position of the fetus). *Progress* in labor is determined by the gradual descent of the presenting part, or change in *station* (the location of the presenting part in the birth canal). Designation of station as "+" or "−" refers to the level in cm below (+) or above (−) the *ischial spines*. *Station 0* is attained when the presenting part has reached the *level* of the ischial *spines*. Station +2, for example, is attained when the presenting part is 2 cm below the spines. When the occiput is at station 0, the vertex is said to be *engaged clinically*. Engagement occurs when the fetal biparietal diameter has passed the plane of the *pelvic inlet*.

Presentation, or lie, is the relation of the long axis of the fetus to the long axis of the mother. It may be either *longitudinal* or *transverse*. With a longitudinal lie the presenting part is either the *head* (*cephalic*) or the *breech*. With a transverse lie the *shoulder* is the presenting part. Cephalic presentations are classified according to the relation of the head to the body of the fetus. When the head is fully *flexed* and the chin contacts the thorax, the *occiput*, or *vertex*, presents. When the neck is fully *extended* and the occiput contacts the back, a *face* presentation results, with the *chin*, or *mentum*, the presenting part. Intermediate conditions include the *sinciput*, in which the *large fontanelle* presents, and the partially extended head, in which the *brow* presents. Sinciput and brow presentations usually convert spontaneously to vertex or face presentations by flexion or extension, respectively, during the course of labor.

Position is the relation of a designated point on the presenting part of the fetus to a designated point in the maternal pelvis. For example, if the *occiput* occupies the right anterior portion of the maternal pelvis, the position is designated ROA or ORA. In the case of a *breech* the designated point is the *sacrum* (as in LST) and in the case of a *face* it is the *chin*, or *mentum* (as in RMA).

During the course of pregnancy painless irregular uterine contractions (Braxton Hicks contractions) increase in intensity and regularity and eventually become true labor pains. The contractions of true labor begin in the lumbar region at intervals of 20 to 30 minutes. At the onset of labor the mucous plug is expelled from the cervical canal.

A normal effective uterine contraction reaches an intensity of 40 to 60 mm Hg. Uterine contractions of an intensity less than 15 mm Hg are ineffective. The latent phase in a primigravida lasts about 8.5 hours and ends when the cervical dilatation is about 2.5 cm. The accelerated phase lasts about two hours and occurs while the cervix dilates from 2.5 to 4 cm. The phase of maximal slope lasts about two hours and occurs while the cervix is dilating from 4 to 9 cm. The phase of deceleration lasts about two hours and occurs during the last centimeter of dilatation of the cervix. The total length of labor in the multigravida is normally several hours shorter than in the primigravida.

During labor the fetal head may be in varying degrees of flexion or extension (habitus or attitude). A fully flexed vertex occurs in about 95% of all deliveries. The fetal head may undergo certain changes in shape to accommodate to the configuration of the maternal pelvis. Molding is a change in shape of the fetal head in labor that is brought about by the forces of labor, the resistance of the bony pelvis, and the loose connections between the fetal skull bones. The head may also undergo lateral flexion (asynclitism). Synclitism exists when the fetal head presents with the sagittal suture midway between the maternal symphysis pubis and the sacral promontory. In anterior asynclitism, the sagittal suture approaches the sacral promontory and the anterior parietal bone of the fetus is the most dependent portion of the head in the birth canal. In posterior asynclitism the sagittal suture approaches the symphysis pubis and the posterior parietal bone is most dependent.

During long labor a caput succedaneum may be formed. In the process the portion of the fetal scalp immediately over the cervical os becomes edematous and may prevent the differentiation of sutures and fontanelles by the examiner. Molding, asynclitism, deflexion, and caput may all lead to an erroneous diagnosis of station, since the head feels lower than it actually is. When the fetal head has negotiated the pelvic outlet and its largest diameter is encircled by the vulvar ring, crowning is said to take place.

Throughout labor the fetal status must be monitored by the recording of heart rate by *stethoscopic* auscultation or *electronic* methods. The maternal status must be monitored by the recording of *vital signs* every 15 minutes, *urinary output,* and the *quality* and *frequency* of uterine *contractions.* Fetal *position* should be ascertained by *abdominal* and *vaginal examination.* When the fetal position or presentation is in doubt, *consultation* is mandatory. *Failure of progress* of labor for *two hours* and detection of a *small pelvis* or a *fetal abnormality* also require *consultation.* The method of *pain control,* analgesia and anesthesia, may affect the progress of labor and the status of the fetus (p. 62).

If no vaginal bleeding is detected, *vaginal examination* should be performed to ascertain *station, cervical dilatation,* and *effacement.* The vaginal or rectal examinations must be repeated under aseptic conditions at appropriate intervals. During the first stage the patient may have an *enema* and a *perineal preparation* as for a surgical procedure. A *large-bore intravenous needle* should be inserted, especially if there is increased likelihood of blood transfusion. The patient should take *nothing by mouth* after the onset of labor. The *bladder* should *not* be *catheterized* unless the patient cannot void or a difficult operative delivery is anticipated. During the *second stage,* as the patient begins to bear down, maternal vital signs and fetal heart rate are *monitored more frequently.* The multipara is often transported to the delivery room when the cervix is 7 to 8 cm dilated, and the primigravida at full dilatation, depending on the rapidity of labor.

The normal *mechanism* of *labor* in a vertex involves: engagement, descent, flexion, internal rotation, extension, external rotation, and expulsion. After the *head* is born the *shoulders* are delivered, followed more or less rapidly by the remainder of the *body.*

The cause of the onset of labor is basically unknown, but important factors may include: release of the progesterone block of myometrial activity, changing relations of oxytocin and oxytocinase, effects of prostaglandins, and fetal endocrine activity. The principal problem in diagnosis of labor is its differentiation from false labor, which unlike true labor is unaccompanied by progressive dilatation of the cervix or increasingly forceful contractions. It can be differentiated from the latent phase of labor with certainty only on retrospective evaluation. The hazards of false labor include maternal exhaustion, apprehension, and premature intervention by the obstetrician.

Diagnosis of presentation and position is made by abdominal palpation, rectal or vaginal examination, auscultation of the location of the fetal heart, sonography, and roentgenography. The breech feels softer than the head, and the back feels larger, smoother, and firmer than the small parts, which are nodular and irregular. If the cephalic prominence is felt on the same side as the small parts, the head is flexed. If the cephalic prominence is on the same side as the back, the head is extended.

The typical obstetric inlet has an anteroposterior diameter of 11.5 cm and a transverse diameter of 13 cm. The plane of least pelvic dimensions in the midpelvis has an anteroposterior diameter of 12 cm and a transverse diameter of 10.5 cm. If the inlet and midpelvis are adequate, it is unlikely that the outlet will cause difficulty in delivery. The normal biparietal diameter of the term fetus is about 9.25 cm and the bitemporal about 8.0 cm. When there is difficulty in engagement in the transverse diameter, the bitemporal diameter is often substituted for the biparietal diameter and extension is the result. In normal circumstances, flexion results in making the suboccipitobregmatic (9.5 cm) rather than the occipitofrontal (11.5 cm) the engaging diameter.

The anterior fontanelle (bregma) is the diamond-shaped junction of the parietal and frontal bones. The posterior fontanelle is the triangular junction of the two parietal bones and the occipital bone.

In certain circumstances x-ray pelvimetry is helpful in deciding the further management of labor. Indications include: clinically contracted inlet or outlet or prominent ischial spines; an unengaged vertex in a primigravida in labor; most cases of breech presentation in a primigravida; a fetus judged to weigh over 4000 g; other malpresentations with a term-sized fetus; previous obstetric complications resulting in difficult forceps deliveries; and failure of progress in labor despite good uterine contractions. X-ray pelvimetry in conjunction with ultrasonic cephalometry usually provides the required information for the diagnosis of cephalopelvic disproportion.

If the membranes rupture during the first stage of labor, the size of the uterine cavity decreases and the pressure of the head directly on the lower uterine segment may improve the efficiency of labor. Immediately after rupture of the membranes a vaginal examination should be done to detect prolapse of the umbilical cord. It is occasionally difficult to know whether the fluid leaking from the vagina is urine or amniotic in origin. Nitrazine paper may be used to detect the alkaline pH that is characteristic of amniotic fluid but not urine. Microscopic examination may be employed to detect fetal epithelial cells, fat globules, and hair, which are normally released into the amniotic fluid.

Fetal monitoring during labor is greatly improved by adding electronic surveillance to clinical methods. In the first stage of labor the fetal heart rate may drop during contractions but rises again to between 120 and 160/min between contractions. Occasionally detection of tachycardia, bradycardia, or irregularity of the fetal heart rate by stethoscope calls attention to the need for more precise electronic monitoring. The combination of abnormalities of the fetal heart rate and passage of meconium is serious. Auscultation of the fetal heart should be even more frequent during the second stage.

Several patterns emerge when simultaneous electronic monitoring of the fetal heart rate and uterine contractions is carried out. When deceleration of the fetal heart rate occurs immediately after the onset of uterine contractions, the pattern known as early deceleration, or Type I dips, results. This pattern should suggest compression of the fetal head and is not an ominous sign. Bradycardia occurring late after the onset of uterine contractions is called late deceleration, or Type II dips. This pattern usually indicates uteroplacental insufficiency. A variable onset of deceleration with respect to the uterine contraction often indicates compression of the umbilical cord.

Type II dips may be caused by maternal hypotension or excessive uterine activity resulting from administration of oxytocin. If correction of maternal hypotension and discontinuation of the oxytocin do not correct the pattern, prompt delivery may be indicated. Variable deceleration is often corrected by repositioning of the mother and administration of oxygen. If these factors do not reverse the pattern, operative delivery may be required to avoid the hazards of prolonged compression of the cord. Analysis of the pH of blood from the fetal scalp may be helpful in deciding the management. Acidosis suggests a more serious degree of fetal compromise (Table 5). The oxytocin challenge test, or contraction stress test, indicates the response of the fetal heart rate to transient reduction in uteroplacental blood flow, and thus fetal oxygenation. A positive test is the occurrence of late deceleration with uterine activity below the level of three to four contractions in ten minutes. The test is considered negative, or normal, when late decelerations are absent at this level of stress. The test usually requires one to two hours.

TABLE 5. Management of Fetal Distress

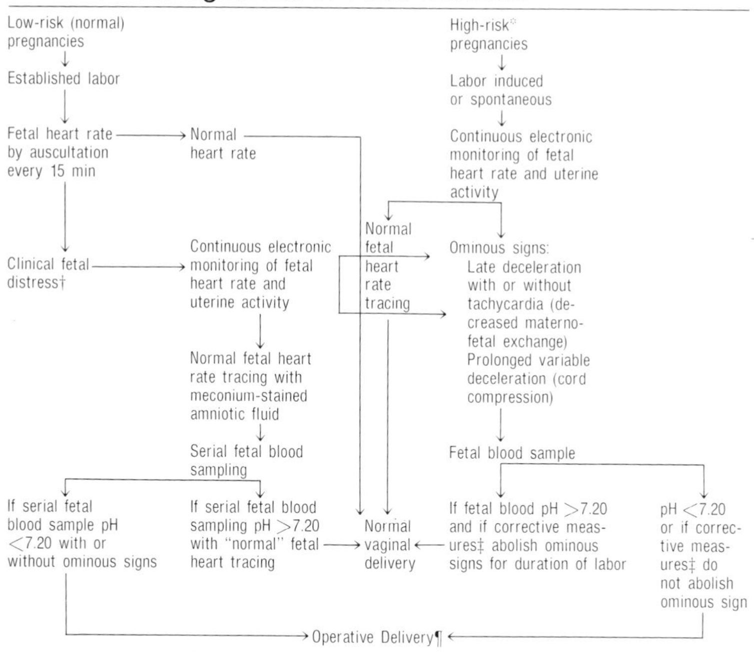

*For example: diabetes, chronic hypertension, preeclampsia, premature labor, and third-trimester bleeding.
†Auscultated fetal heart rate >160 or <120/min or meconium staining of amniotic fluid.
‡Change in maternal position to alleviate maternal hypotension or cord-compression. Decrease or discontinuation of intravenous oxytocin infusion to alleviate uterine hyperactivity.
¶Anticipate birth of depressed newborn and have available obstetric or pediatric personnel skilled in direct resuscitation.

Nonstressed monitoring has been used recently as another means of assessing intrauterine well-being. The baseline and variability of the fetal heart rate and the occurrence of accelerations of the rate with fetal movement are taken as indications of the integrity of the reflexes controlling cardiac rate. The pattern is considered reactive if the baseline rate is between 120 and 150 beats per minute, the baseline variability is 10 beats per minute or more, and at least five fetal movements accompanied by accelerations of 15 beats per minute or more occur during a period of 20 minutes. The advantages of nonstressed monitoring include the virtual absence of contraindications, the avoidance of drugs, and the short period of only 30 minutes required for its completion.

In both stressed and nonstressed monitoring the prediction of fetal compromise is less certain than the confirmation of fetal well-being. These tests must be used in conjunction with measurements of estriol, indices of fetal maturity, and most important, relevant clinical data in deciding the need for delivery.

Amnioscopy is a technique for evaluation of the color and turbidity of the amniotic fluid by means of transcervical examination through an endoscope. Meconium staining is associated with a lower Apgar score and a higher perinatal mortality. It is used more often in countries other than the United States and is valuable principally in conjunction with other tests of fetal well-being.

The level of alpha-fetoprotein in the amniotic fluid increases in the presence of severe fetal distress or impending fetal death. A marked elevation of the level of alpha-fetoprotein is found in association with anencephaly and other open neural tube defects.

Most fetuses *engage* in the *occiput transverse* position and deliver as *occipitoanteriors*. In a typical labor the head is born by *extension* over the perineum, followed by *external rotation* back to the transverse or anterior position. The patient should be instructed not to bear down before the second stage.

Delivery is most safely accomplished *spontaneously* or by *low forceps* extraction. *Excessive* or *premature* administration of *anesthesia* results in the need for *more difficult forceps* deliveries.

The head should be delivered between contractions. During spontaneous delivery the obstetrician should cover the patient's anus with a towel and apply upward pressure on the chin through the perineum. The obstetrician's other hand should be used to control the egress of the head by gentle pressure on the occiput. As soon as the head is delivered, loops of cord should be removed from the infant's neck. Delivery of the shoulders should be delayed until they are in the anteroposterior diameter of the outlet. One shoulder should be delivered at a time. The rest of the body ordinarily follows with ease. In normal circumstances, the newborn should be suspended by its feet below the level of the placenta to allow transfusion of placental blood.

The *third stage* of labor comprises *separation* and *expulsion* of the placenta. Its successful spontaneous termination depends primarily on *uterine activity*. After the placenta separates, the shape of the uterus changes from *discoid* to *globular* and the top of the uterus is felt at a somewhat *higher* level. At the same time there is a *gush of blood* and a *lengthening of the cord*, which yields when slight traction is applied. *Uterine bleeding* after expulsion is *controlled* by occlusion of blood vessels by sustained *uterine contraction*.

The *placenta* should be *routinely inspected* for completeness and the *birth canal* should be examined for *injuries*. A *missing placental cotyledon* or a *torn vessel* on the chorionic surface indicates *retention* of a placental *fragment* within the uterus.

The vital signs of the mother and the uterine tone should be *monitored* for at least *one hour post partum*. The patient should remain in the *recovery room* for *two to three hours* before being returned to her room.

The average blood loss during normal vaginal delivery without episiotomy is about *300 ml*. The blood loss is often greater than it appears without accurate measurement. Loss of blood of *500 ml* or more is considered *postpartum hemorrhage* (p. 97).

The placenta is best delivered as soon as possible after it has separated, with care taken to remove all the membranes as well. In the presence of excessive bleeding or after 30 minutes in the third stage, it is wisest to remove the placenta manually under appropriate anesthesia. No traction should be applied to the cord until the placenta has separated. Premature or forceful traction may result in inversion of the uterus, a serious accident that may lead to shock and may require hysterectomy.

Many regimens for the administration of oxytocic agents are employed. One entirely satisfactory method is the addition of 10 units of oxytocin to the intravenous infusion. The oxytocin should not be given in a single intravenous push. An alternative method is the intramuscular administration of 10 units of oxytocin immediately after delivery of the placenta. To avoid trapping of the placenta, it is wisest to defer the administration of oxytocin until after the completion of the third stage, although some obstetricians use it at the time of delivery of the shoulders. Some oxytocic regimens include 0.2 mg of methylergonovine maleate intravenously or intramuscularly after delivery of the placenta. Ergot derivatives are not recommended, however, in the presence of hypertension or preeclampsia.

When uterine atony is anticipated, as in cases of overdistension of the uterus or prolonged labor, it is best to keep the oxytocin infusion running for several hours after the third stage.

The problems of obstetric anesthesia differ from those of anesthesia in general because of the *altered maternal physiologic* functions in pregnancy, the presence of the *fetus* (which is particularly *sensitive* to *anesthetic agents*), alterations in *maternal homeostasis* resulting from anesthesia, and often the *emergency* during which obstetric anesthesia must be administered. In particular, the changes in maternal *respiratory* and *cardiovascular function* tend to alter the *speed* of *induction* of *inhalation* anesthesia; the *diminished volumes* of *spinal canal* and *epidural spaces* necessitate *smaller amounts* of *local* anesthetic agents to achieve a similar level of anesthesia; furthermore, there is the effect of the *diminished venous return*, which results from the *compression* of the *inferior vena cava* by the gravid uterus (supine hypotensive syndrome). The *drop in peripheral resistance* and the venous dilatation secondary to sympathetic blockage resulting from major regional anesthesia, in combination with inferior vena cava compression, may cause life-threatening *hypotension*. Finally, all general and local anesthetic agents, barbiturates, tranquilizers, and narcotics *cross the placenta*. Analgesia may be achieved during labor and delivery by means of narcotics and other types of analgesic agents, regional blocks, or general anesthetics.

General anesthesia must be *avoided* when the patient's *stomach is full*, unless *intubation* can be promptly carried out. *Analgesia* (such as 100 mg of meperidine) should be *withheld until labor* is clearly established, and *regional blocks* should not be performed *until the cervix is at least 4 to 5 cm* dilated. The *choice* of anesthetic agent depends on the *availability* of the technique and the *skills* of the personnel. It should be tailored to the type of delivery and the desires of the patient whenever possible. For example, a low *forceps* or a *normal spontaneous delivery* of a multipara can often be effected by *analgesia* and a *pudendal* block. A *forceps* delivery of a *primigravida*, however, may often be managed best by *lumbar epidural, caudal,* or *low subarachnoid* (*saddle*) block. Deliveries that require extensive *intrauterine manipulations* should be conducted with maximal uterine *relaxation*, such as is provided by *halothane* or *ether*.

Analgesia during labor is most often accomplished by means of narcotic agents. These drugs rapidly cross the placental barrier and may affect the fetus' respiratory center. The intravenous and intramuscular routes of administration are both acceptable. Narcotics are often used in combination with tranquilizers because of a possible synergistic effect. Barbiturates, unless used in anesthetic amounts, are not analgesic but reduce anxiety. Tranquilizers alone are often helpful during early first stage of labor when anxiety rather than pain is the principal problem. Scopolamine in large doses and in combination with narcotics causes amnesia, but also excitation, which may be difficult to control. Inhalation anesthetic agents such as nitrous oxide, methoxyflurane, and trichloroethylene may be used in subanesthetic concentrations to obtund painful sensations during labor and delivery. Inhalation analgesia may be used in conjunction with narcotics. The patient must be carefully watched and protected from unnecessarily deep anesthetic levels.

Anesthesia remains a major cause of maternal mortality in the United States (p. 120), where general anesthesia is still the most popular method for achieving pain relief during delivery.

General anesthesia, however, is responsible for most of the deaths attributable to anesthesia; 50% are attributed to aspiration of gastric contents. This form of anesthesia must be approached with the greatest care if the patient has eaten within six hours of the onset of labor. Even if six hours have elapsed, however, the stomach is not necessarily empty. All patients in labor must therefore be considered as having full stomachs. Aspiration of gastric contents is often fatal. All inhalation anesthetic agents, with the exception of nitrous oxide, depress the myometrium and can abolish uterine contractions. Ether and halothane have been the most popular agents for this purpose when the obstetrician needs uterine relaxation.

The purpose of regional anesthesia is to block sensations arising from the cervix, uterus, and perineum. The pain pathways during the first stage of labor involve visceral afferent nerve fibers that arise from the uterus and cervix. The pains of the second stage of labor arise from somatic afferent receptors and fibers in the vulva and perineum and travel by way of the inferior hemorrhoidal nerve, the labial nerve, and the dorsal nerve of the clitoris. These nerves join to form the pudendal nerves.

Paracervical blocks administered in the vaginal fornices block pain impulses at the level of the uterine plexus. Lumbar epidural and caudal blocks interrupt pain sensations in the epidural space before the nerve's entrance into the spinal canal. Subarachnoid anesthesia blocks the nerves in the spinal canal where they bathe directly in the cerebrospinal fluid. Pudendal blocks interrupt only pain sensations arising from the perineum and vulva and are useful only in the second stage of labor. Paracervical anesthesia does not block the sacral segments and therefore does not relieve pain arising from the perineum. Spinal, lumbar epidural, and caudal blocks may be used to interrupt painful sensations from the uterus, cervix, and perineum.

Toxic reactions to local anesthetics are most often related to overdosage of circulating local anesthetic agents. This result can occur after careless use of any of the techniques mentioned except spinal anesthesia. The high incidence of hypotension that can occur following any major block resulting in sympathetic blockade is important. Therapeutic measures must be taken immediately if hypotension develops. The steps include lifting the uterus off the inferior vena cava or placing the patient on her left side; rapid hydration of the patient with 1 liter of a balanced salt solution; and vasopressors administered intravenously if the previous measures do not return the pressure to normal levels. Since the drop in blood pressure must be quickly noted and treated, major regional blocks must be preceded by: the application of a blood pressure cuff that is to be left in place, constant monitoring of vital signs, and the establishment of a dependable means of intravenous medication (intravenous cannulas or catheters).

Less local anesthetic is required to achieve a given level of anesthesia in late pregnancy than in the nonpregnant state. Hypotension resulting from regional blocks must be treated to maintain a maternal systolic pressure of at least 100 mm Hg. Lower pressures may impair perfusion of the intervillous space and result in fetal hypoxia, hypercarbia, and acidosis.

Complications resulting from major regional blocks such as spinals and epidurals include overdosage, with central nervous system impairment and convulsions; chemical and septic meningitis; constrictive arachnoiditis; and postpuncture headaches. The complications are generally preventable.

Regional anesthesia is preferred over other forms of anesthesia because the complications arising from these methods are preventable or treatable, and they appear to be less dangerous to the fetus. Spinal, caudal, and lumbar epidural anesthesia are contraindicated, however, if: the patient is hypovolemic or suffers from a complication that is accompanied by blood loss; the patient is hypotensive; there is skin infection at the site of puncture; there is an active neurologic disorder; the patient is receiving anticoagulants; the patient refuses the procedure; and the physician lacks the experience or adequate equipment for administration, monitoring, and resuscitation.

The need for highly skilled physicians to administer major regional blocks or general anesthesia has not been met. The safest, easiest way of achieving pain relief during parturition thus appears to be the careful administration of small doses of narcotics and tranquilizers during labor, followed by a pudendal block and subanesthetic concentrations of general anesthetic agents for delivery.

General anesthetic agents in obstetrics may be employed for three purposes: in subanesthetic concentrations for analgesia; general anesthesia of a degree sufficient for delivery or cesarean section; as myometrial relaxants for intrauterine manipulations such as breech extraction or version and extraction, replacement of an inverted uterus, relaxation of tetanic contractions, and removal of a retained placenta. Because of the danger of aspiration of gastric contents, endotracheal intubation is always indicated when general anesthesia is administered. Endotracheal intubation can be performed with the patient awake after topical anesthesia of the pharynx and larynx or with the patient asleep after the rapid administration of a fast-acting barbiturate, followed immediately by a muscle relaxant. Cricoid pressure should be maintained to compress the esophagus and prevent regurgitation. Pressure should be maintained until the endotracheal tube cuff has been inflated and the airway protected.

Aspiration of gastric contents can cause death by two different mechanisms. First, obstruction of the airway renders the capillary-alveolar gas exchange impossible. Second, if the pH of the gastric juice is below 2.5, contact with the respiratory tree often results in bronchospasm, pulmonary edema, and death. If the patient survives the immediate injury, severe atelectasis and chemical pneumonitis may ensue. The treatment consists in quickly clearing the airway by suction, administration of 100% oxygen by means of an endotracheal tube, treating the bronchospasm with isoproterenol, steroids in high doses, and broad-spectrum antibiotics.

The first and most important factor in the prevention of aspiration pneumonitis is the awareness that every parturient is at high risk. It has been recommended that patients receive oral antacids throughout labor. Although these drugs do not protect against aspiration of solid material, they lower significantly the risk of damage to the lung by acidic fluids.

The use of vasopressors for the treatment of hypotension secondary to major regional blocks is based on their ability to increase venous return by activating adrenergic receptors and therefore causing a rise in peripheral resistance and venous constriction. Furthermore, they can increase venous return by activating beta-adrenergic receptors and cause an increase in cardiac inotropism and chronotropism. Some vasopressors do both. In obstetrics the use of alpha-adrenergic stimulants such as methoxamine is contraindicated because the rise in maternal blood pressure is accompanied by uterine arterial vasoconstriction, diminished perfusion of the intervillous space, and resulting aggravation of fetal distress. Agents that have mainly beta-adrenergic receptor-activating effects are preferred. The principal agent is ephedrine. In preeclampsia-eclampsia, vasopressors must be used in smaller doses because of the increased adrenergic receptor sensitivity. Ergot derivatives must not be used after vasopressors have been administered. There is a synergistic effect between these two types of medications that may lead to lethal hypertension.

The rate at which an inhalation agent will affect a fetus is difficult to predict because it is dependent upon many variables involving the mother, placenta, and fetus. An intravenous anesthetic agent such as thiopental, however, rapidly reaches the fetus. After an injection of thiopental, equilibrium between mother and fetus is reached in less than two minutes. Thereafter the fetus continues to accumulate thiopental. As the concentration of thiopental in the mother diminishes, however, as a result of redistribution to various spaces, so does that in the fetus. The concentration in the umbilical vein is always higher than in the umbilical artery. It is therefore impossible to deliver the baby before equilibrium is reached. The anesthesiologist should not hurry the obstetrician, but the obstetrician should work with careful speed.

When spinal anesthesia is to be administered it is important to be proficient in the use of 25-gauge or 26-gauge spinal needles. The incidence of postpuncture headaches is directly related to the size of the rent made in the dura in the course of the administration of a spinal block. During administration of an epidural block, a small test dose must be given to ascertain whether the subarachnoid space has been inadvertently entered. The accidental subarachnoid injection of the usual doses of local anesthetics used for epidural anesthesia may result in a very high or total spinal block. Resuscitation equipment and drugs must be on hand at all times.

Normal Puerperium

The puerperium is the period of time, usually about *six weeks,* from delivery until the *genital tract* returns to the *normal nonpregnant condition.* After an uncomplicated spontaneous delivery the multiparous patient may often be discharged as early as 24 hours post partum. Primigravidas and all patients with episiotomies usually require a stay of several days in the hospital post partum. In all cases the patient should be allowed to *ambulate* and to use the *bathroom* as soon after delivery as she can comfortably do so. She should be encouraged to *empty* her *bladder* at least every eight hours to avoid overdistension, which may predispose to infection. A mild *cathartic* may be prescribed after 48 hours if the patient has not moved her bowels. *Codeine* (0.06 g) and *aspirin* (0.6 g) may be prescribed for *afterpains.* These pains are more common in the multipara but usually subside by 48 hours post partum. The *perineum* should be kept *clean* during the puerperium. Painful sites of *episiotomy* or *lacerations* may be treated symptomatically with *sitz baths* and a *heat lamp.* If the *lochia* (vaginal discharge during the puerperium) are particularly *bloody, methergine* (methylergonovine maleate) may be prescribed in 6 doses of 0.2 mg at four-hour intervals.

Postpartum *chills* are *common* but not necessarily indicative of infection. The temperature should be recorded every six hours for the first 24 hours at least. A *slight elevation* (rarely over 100.4° F) is *common* after a difficult labor or delivery, but it usually falls to normal within 24 hours. A *sustained* elevation or a *rising temperature* suggests *infection* (p. 119).

In certain situations in which *Rh-isoimmunization* is thought to have been initiated, *anti-D globulin* (RhoGAM) should be given shortly after delivery (p. 104). Since the patient may *ovulate* very *soon* after delivery, *contraceptive* advice should be given while she is still in the hospital and repeated at the time of the postpartum checkup. Coitus is best avoided until all discomfort has subsided and all wounds have healed.

The *postpartum examination* usually takes place between *four* and *six weeks* after delivery. At that time the physical examination should include measurement of the *blood pressure* and *hematocrit,* examination of the *breasts, abdomen,* and *pelvis*, and a *Papanicolaou smear* if it has not been done in the preceding six months.

Colostrum is secreted for about *two days* after delivery, at which time *lactation* begins. The milk attains a stable composition after the first month. If the mother does not intend to breast feed the baby, *lactation may be suppressed by steroids* early in the puerperium. One good method is *estradiol valerate* and *testosterone enanthate* (Deladumone) in a single intramuscular injection of 4 ml. Treatment with steroids after *lactogenesis* is initiated will not suppress the process. When no drugs are used, painful *engorgement* of the breasts normally *disappears* within *36* to *48* hours. Symptomatic relief of engorgement is provided by supportive *binders, ice bags, fluids* by mouth, and *analgesics*. The mammary ducts usually fill with milk between the second and fifth days post partum. *Suckling* and the administration of *oxytocin* stimulate the *let-down* of milk. The obstetrician must be aware that many *drugs* administered to the nursing mother may be *transferred* to the *newborn* in the *milk*.

Prolactin (LTH, lactogenic hormone, mammotropic hormone) is required for lactogenesis (initiation of the secretion of milk) and galactopoiesis (continuation of secretion of milk). The hormone also serves to maintain the cholesterol precursors in the ovary for the secretion of steroids.

Prolactin is a polypeptide similar in structure to growth hormone. It is secreted by acidophils of the anterior pituitary. Its release is promoted by thyrotropic releasing hormone (TRH) and inhibited by prolactin inhibiting factor (PIF) of the hypothalamus. PIF and GnRH are generally released and repressed together. Thus, when LH and FSH are secreted, prolactin is inhibited. An exception occurs during the midcycle gonadotropic surge, when there is also marked release of prolactin, presumably an action of TRH. During lactation and occasionally in women receiving phenothiazine tranquilizers, both PIF and GnRH are repressed, with resulting anovulation. Lactation may be induced via the central nervous system from stimulation of the breast or psychological factors associated with nursing.

By the tenth postpartum day the uterus has descended into the pelvis, that is, has regressed to the size of a three months' gestation. During the puerperium the weight of the uterus decreases from 1000 g to 100 g. In this process, known as involution, individual myometrial cells decrease in size. The endometrial lining is usually restored after several weeks as the placental site regresses. Involution of the placental site is normally complete by six weeks post partum. Interference with this process may result in late postpartum hemorrhage (p. 120). The lochia gradually change from red (lochia rubra) to pinkish or yellowish (lochia serosa) to whitish (lochia alba) as the proportions of erythrocytes, leukocytes, and decidual debris change. Lochial discharge normally continues for about four weeks to as long as eight weeks post partum.

The first normal menstrual period usually occurs between four and eight weeks post partum and is often heavy. The patient may ovulate, however, as early as the second or third day post partum. Lactation may delay or suppress menstruation, but does not in itself provide adequate contraception.

During the puerperium a diuresis resulting in a loss of about five pounds takes place between the second and fifth postpartum days. The loss of fluid may be even greater in preeclampsia (p. 99).

Leukocytosis immediately after labor may rise to as high as 30,000. The hemoglobin and hematocrit may vary somewhat during the postpartum period, but normally do not fall below the values before delivery unless the blood loss has been considerable. At one week post partum the blood volume is normally back to the level before pregnancy.

The Neonate

As soon as the *head* is delivered, the infant's *nose* and *throat* should be *aspirated* with a bulb syringe to clear the airway. During delivery the infant should be *suspended* by the *feet* above the obstetrician's lap but held *below* the level of the *perineum* to facilitate *transfusion* of *placental blood*. The *cord* of a normal infant should be allowed to *stop pulsating* before it is clamped. Double clamping is best performed about 4 cm from the umbilicus. During the period immediately after delivery the infant should be kept *warm* before transfer to the nursery. *Handling* of the newborn, particularly the premature, should be *minimized*. The newborn's *eyes* should be treated with *penicillin* ointment or *silver nitrate* (1% solution) to prevent gonorrheal ophthalmia.

The *Apgar score* should be recorded at *1 minute* and *5 minutes* after birth to permit objective transfer of information among obstetrician, anesthesiologist, and pediatrician (Table 6). Apgar scores of *0* to *3* denote a severely *depressed* infant; scores of *4* to *6* suggest a *fair* general condition; and scores of *7* or *above* indicate a baby in *good* condition. All newborns with scores of 0 to 3 and many with scores of 4 to 6 need *resuscitation*.

Immediate erection of the penis and urination are usually signs of a healthy infant. The newborn's *footprints* should be obtained and *identification bracelets* applied as soon after delivery as possible.

The *pediatrician* should be *forewarned* of any *complications* during pregnancy, labor, or delivery and should be *informed*

TABLE 6. Apgar Score

SIGN	0	1	2
Heart rate	Absent	Slow (Below 100)	Over 100
Respiratory effort	Absent	Weak cry; hypoventilation	Good effort; strong cry
Muscle tone	Limp	Some flexion of extremities	Active motion; extremities well flexed
Reflex irritability (Response to stimulation) of skin of feet	No response	Some motion (Grimace)	Crying and active
Color	Blue, pale	Body pink; extremities blue	Completely pink

about any *drugs* that the mother may have taken. If the baby is *jaundiced* soon after birth, it may require an *exchange transfusion*. In such a case the umbilical *cord* should be left *long* and a *pediatric consultation* obtained immediately.

The *placenta* should be *examined* carefully to see whether it is *intact* and to detect *gross lesions*. A cross section of the *cord* should be inspected to detect the *absence* of *one umbilical artery*, an anomaly that is found in 1% of infants and is often associated with other congenital malformations.

Circumcision of the newborn male is recommended by most American obstetricians. Among its advantages are improved penile *hygiene* and *prevention* of *penile carcinoma*. Good technique and several new instruments ensure the safety of the procedure. The operation should be *deferred* in *premature* or *sick* infants and those with a *bleeding tendency* or a *penile anomaly* such as *hypospadias*. The procedure should not be performed immediately after delivery, but rather a few days later, after the infant has been observed to remain well.

The delivery room must have immediately available at all times equipment for resuscitation, including endotracheal tubes and laryngoscopes, umbilical vein catheters, oxygen, and suction devices.

A newborn may be incapable of maintaining normal respiration for several reasons including: intrauterine asphyxia or inadequate placental exchange, prematurity, congenital anomalies, drugs administered to the mother, trauma during labor or delivery, and anemia secondary to blood group incompatibility.

Intrauterine hypoxia or asphyxia may result from maternal disorders such as diabetes, hypertension, hypotension, preeclampsia, and renal disease. Additional factors include premature separation of the placenta, compression of the umbilical cord, and tetanic uterine contractions. Prematurity is associated with incomplete development of the lung and inadequate production of surfactant, leading to alveolar instability and predisposition to respiratory distress syndrome. Narcotics, barbiturates, and all anesthetic agents administered to the mother may depress the fetal central nervous and cardiovascular systems.

In resuscitating an infant the first step is rapid clearing of the airway. The second step is administration of oxygen by positive pressure ventilation. Resuscitation by bag and mask connected to a source of oxygen will permit the administration of 30 to 100% oxygen, depending on the type of equipment used. In performing positive pressure ventilation, the infant's head should be elevated and extended without exerting any pressure on soft tissues. When the babies are severely ill and when the results of the efforts at resuscitation are poor, oral endotracheal intubation under direct vision with a laryngoscope should be performed, but only by personnel trained in this technique. Improper or premature use of endotracheal intubation may result in further jeopardizing the baby by delaying the administration of oxygen and prolonging asphyxia. Careful external cardiac massage is mandatory if the baby suffers from severe bradycardia and appears pale.

Hypoxemia rapidly leads to anaerobic metabolism and acidosis, which should be counteracted by the administration of 4.5 to 9 mEq/kg of sodium bicarbonate. This drug should be administered into the fetal circulation by means of a catheter introduced into the umbilical vein or one of the umbilical arteries. Fetal blood pH and base excess should be checked repeatedly and, if necessary, compensated by further administration of sodium bicarbonate.

Narcotic antagonists should be administered only if respiratory depression can be clearly attributed to prior administration of narcotics to the mother. Asphyxia or hypoxia results in delayed closure or in reopening of the ductus arteriosus, pulmonary hypertension, decreased pulmonary blood flow, loss of alveolar surfactant, unstable alveoli, acidosis, and cardiovascular depression. All these factors, if untreated, increase hypoxia and create a vicious cycle.

UNIT III

Obstetric Abnormalities

Spontaneous Abortion

The most common causes of vaginal bleeding in women in the reproductive age group are related to complications of pregnancy. Abortion is the termination of pregnancy *before fetal viability,* or when the fetus weighs *less than 500* g. Abortion may be *spontaneous* (occurring through natural causes) or *induced* (by mechanical or medicinal means). Most spontaneous abortions occur in the *second* or *third month* of gestation. Induced abortion may be *medically indicated* or *elective.* Local laws rather than medical grounds determine whether an abortion is *legal* or *criminal.*

Spontaneous abortions occur in *more than 10%* of all pregnancies. The true rate is probably closer to 20%, for many of the earliest abortions are *not recognized* by the patient. The *cause* of spontaneous abortion is *unknown* in the majority of cases, although *blighted ova* and other less profound fetal *genetic abnormalities* (proved by chromosomal analysis) may be detected in a significant proportion of conceptuses. *Local* and *systemic maternal disorders* and *environmental factors* may all be operative. Maternal diseases include acute and chronic *infections* (such as toxoplasmosis), chronic *wasting diseases,* and *endocrinopathies* (particularly thyroid dysfunction). Local factors include *anomalies of the reproductive tract, myomas,* or *incompetence of the cervix.* External environmental factors include *trauma, radiation,* and *cytotoxic drugs.*

Threatened abortion is diagnosed on the basis of any *vaginal* bleeding in the *first twenty weeks* of pregnancy. *Only half* of all cases of threatened abortion will *progress* to abortion regardless of treatment. Diagnosis requires a *gynecologic examination* to rule out other causes of vaginal bleeding, such as cervical polyps and neoplasms as well as injuries to the lower genital tract. With threatened abortion the uterine bleeding may be accompanied by *cramps* and *backache,* the *uterine size is consistent* with the *menstrual history,* and the *cervix is not dilated.* If the *pain* accompanying uterine bleeding is *severe, other complications* of pregnancy must be ruled out, such as ectopic pregnancy and twisted ovarian cyst.

Treatment of threatened abortion is *conservative,* namely, mild sedation and a *few days of bedrest.* Longer periods are not justified, for abortion cannot be forestalled by further bedrest. There is no drug therapy of proven effectiveness. When threatened abortion progresses to *incomplete abortion, part of the product of conception is passed.* Usually a portion of the placenta is *retained* and the incompletely emptied uterus continues to bleed. *Hemorrhage* may be slight or sufficient to produce shock. Abortion is usually *preceded by fetal death* and pathologic examination generally reveals necrosis and hemorrhage in the decidua. The most effective treatment of incomplete abortion is *curettage* (suction or sharp), with *oxytocin* employed in the *larger uteri* (10 to 12 weeks' size or larger). An *intravenous infusion* should be started; in the presence of moderate or severe bleeding *blood* should be crossmatched and available. Complications (more common with induced abortion) include *sepsis* and *shock. Septic abortion* is a leading cause of *maternal mortality* in the United States.

In cases of *complete abortion* the *entire product* of conception is passed. Bleeding is usually minimal and *no treatment* is ordinarily required.

In cases of *missed abortion* the fetus dies but is retained in utero for *more than two months.* Diagnosis is made on the basis of *regression of signs* of pregnancy. The uterus should be evacuated as soon as the fetus is known to be dead. Early missed abortion may often be managed by intravenous oxytocin followed by curettage. Later abortions may require *intraamniotic injections* of hypertonic solutions.

Habitual abortion is defined as *three or more consecutive spontaneous abortions.* Known causes include uterine anomalies, incompetence of the cervix, inadequate corpus luteum, hypothyroidism, vascular and renal maternal diseases, and immunologic incompatibilities between the parents.

Since half of all threatened abortions fail to progress to frank abortion, any treatment will have a 50% chance of success. Progestin therapy has not been proved effective; it may, furthermore, cause retention of the products of conception and possible masculinization of the genitalia of the female fetus. One quarter to one half of all abortuses will have chromosomal anomalies such as trisomy and polyploidy.

Threatened abortion becomes imminent when the cervix

continues to dilate, usually in conjunction with an increase in abdominal pain. The abortion is considered inevitable when the membranes rupture through a dilated cervix. Patients with imminent and inevitable abortions should be hospitalized and the abortions completed.

An unusual complication of a missed abortion is hypofibrinogenemia, which ordinarily does not occur until five weeks or more after fetal death. The retained fetus occasionally calcifies to form a lithopedion.

Late abortions occurring in the second trimester may be caused by placental abnormalities and maternal diseases such as chronic hypertension. Syphilis may be a cause of late abortion (after the fourth month). Late abortions usually have no discernible cause; they resemble premature deliveries rather than early abortions in the relatively slight bleeding and the moderately severe pain.

The incompetent os is a cause of habitual midtrimester abortion that is not common but is amenable to surgical treatment. It is diagnosed by a history of signs and symptoms that appear in a sequence different from that of the usual incomplete abortion. In the case of incompetent os, the painless, bloodless dilatation of the cervix is followed by rupture of the membranes and then abortion. The pregnancy may be saved by the timely placement of a suture around the internal os. If the pregnancy is carried to term, a cesarean section may be performed or the suture may be cut.

Induced abortions, particularly those performed outside the hospital, may be complicated by hemorrhage, sepsis, acute renal failure, and bacteremic shock. Treatment includes massive antibiotics, scrupulous regulation of fluids and electrolytes to tide the patient over the oliguric phase, and removal of necrotic foci that may be a source of toxins. Nephrotoxic antibiotics must be employed with great caution in patients with impaired renal function. Roentgenograms of the abdomen should be obtained to rule out a foreign body in the peritoneal cavity (perforation of the uterus) or free gas under the diaphragm. Endotoxic shock complicating abortion leads to a high maternal mortality.

Abortion may be induced legally for medical (for example, cardiac, renal, and psychiatric) indications or electively, according to local statutes. Medical indications may be maternal (to preserve the life or health of the mother) or fetal (to prevent abnormalities, as with rubella, or genetic defects, as indicated by amniocentesis.) Before 1973 the legal status of abortion in the United States was chaotic. Techniques, with indications and contraindications for each, are discussed in Unit 7.

Very early abortions (before six weeks) and late abortions (after the sixteenth to twentieth weeks) may be complete. The usual abortion (between the eighth and twelfth weeks), however, is usually incomplete, requiring a curettage. In spontaneous abortion many of the villi may show hydropic change.

Trauma is not a common etiologic factor in abortion. To prove a traumatic cause it must be shown that bleeding and abortion occur shortly after the trauma and that there is no abnormality of the conceptus. Habitual abortion requires careful investigation. In addition to a thorough history and physical examination, a minimal investigation includes a chest film, complete blood count, serologic test for syphilis, protein-bound iodine, glucose tolerance test, hysterogram, measurement of basal body temperature, endometrial biopsy, and progesterone assay.

Septic abortion usually results from instrumental or chemical interference. Uterine perforation, bacterial shock, and hemolysis may be associated. The prominent pathogens were formerly *streptococci* and *staphylococci*, which produced bacteremia. The principal offenders now are gram-negative bacilli (*E. coli* and related organisms), which may produce endotoxic shock, with hypotension, oliguria, and occasionally disseminated intravascular coagulation. Septic abortion caused by pathogenic *clostridia* may produce, in addition, hemolysis and jaundice. The treatment comprises massive antibiotics and attempts to maintain renal function and normal blood pressure. The patient may present with a foul purulent discharge, a boggy tender uterus, and temperature spikes. Prompt curettage to remove necrotic foci is indicated, except in the presence of extrauterine spread (parametritis).

Hypovolemia must be corrected and central venous pressure monitored to avoid overhydration. Metabolic acidosis must be corrected. Endotoxic shock should be suspected whenever hypotension and oliguria are not promptly reversed by intravenous fluids and blood transfusions. Corticosteroids are often given in the face of an inadequate response to fluids, blood, and antibiotics. The blood pressure must be maintained to assure renal perfusion, although the roles of vasoconstrictors and vasodilators are still somewhat controversial. Pressor amines are often given in the presence of warm, dry skin, and vasodilators in the presence of cold, clammy extremities. Mannitol may be used in an attempt to produce diuresis. The role of heparin in preventing or treating intravascular coagulation in cases of infected septic abortion is still controversial. If necrotic foci in the uterus are not accessible to curettage or if there is evidence of uterine perforation, laparotomy and possible hysterectomy may be required as lifesaving measures. The successful management of endotoxic shock depends upon early consultation with the dialysis team and prompt efforts to prevent permanent renal damage.

Ectopic Pregnancy

Pregnancy in any location other than the *body of the uterus* is considered *ectopic*. The vast majority of ectopic pregnancies occur in the *oviduct*. The diagnosis must be considered in any patient of reproductive age with *menstrual irregularity, vaginal spotting, or abdominal pain*. Ectopic pregnancy may be caused by any factor that *retards the passage* of the fertilized egg from ovary to endometrium. The most common cause is *salpingitis*, untreated or inadequately treated. An *adnexal mass* strengthens the diagnosis. *Rupture*, which usually occurs at about eight to ten weeks' gestation, may be heralded by severe *abdominal pain, cervical tenderness, syncope, a drop in hematocrit,* and *shock*.

Hemoperitoneum may often be diagnosed by culdocentesis, although there is a significant possibility of false-negative and false-positive taps. Culdoscopy, laparoscopy, and colpotomy are more time-consuming but more reliable. Pregnancy tests based on hCG are often misleading (false-positive and false-negative). Specific radioimmunoassays for the beta subunit of hCG or radioreceptor assays will minimize the likelihood of false-neg-

Diff Dx.
Appx.
PID
Rupture cyst

ative tests. If there is any doubt about the diagnosis, *laparotomy* is indicated.

The differential diagnosis, which is that of the *acute abdomen* in a woman of reproductive years, includes appendicitis, pelvic inflammatory disease, rupture of a follicle or corpus luteum cyst, and even threatened intrauterine abortion. The primary treatment is *surgical*, with replacement of fluids and blood as soon as possible. The usual procedure is *salpingectomy* and *cornual resection* with no elective surgical procedures at that time.

Tubal gestation appears to have become more common in the last ten years, now occurring once in about 150 pregnancies. The intrauterine device is now believed to cause an absolute increase in the number of oviductal and ovarian pregnancies rather than just an increase in the ratio of ectopic to intrauterine pregnancies. The uterus usually grows at a normal rate for about six to eight weeks and a decidual reaction (without trophoblastic tissue) is commonly found in the endometrium. Any factor that interferes with the function of the fimbriae or causes strictures or adhesions of the tubal wall may predispose to ectopic pregnancy. Operations on the oviduct have become increasingly important etiologic factors.

The termination of the gestation depends largely on the location. Pregnancies in the ampulla, particularly the distal portion, frequently abort with minimal signs. Pregnancies in the isthmus usually rupture into the peritoneal cavity or between the leaves of the broad ligament. Rupture of a pregnancy in the interstitial portion of the tube may be rapidly followed by shock. The resulting hemoperitoneum often causes shoulder pain. Rupture is sometimes precipitated by a Valsalva maneuver, as with straining at stool.

The clinical picture of ectopic pregnancy usually includes a normal temperature, and a normal or only moderately elevated white count. The classic triad of amenorrhea, vaginal bleeding, and pain occurs in only 25% of cases. None of the individual signs occurs in more than 75% of cases and the accuracy of diagnosis does not exceed 80%.

Conservative surgical treatment (expression of the pregnancy from the tube) is occasionally attempted in a nullipara with no adnexa on the opposite side. In a multipara with no adnexa on the other side hysterectomy is occasionally justified in the absence of an acute surgical emergency.

Primary abdominal and ovarian pregnancies are rare. Most are secondary to tubal gestation. An abdominal pregnancy is characterized by easy palpation of the fetal parts, abnormal presentations (often transverse lie), and radiologic evidence of a fetus that appears to be overlying the maternal vertebral column. Although the fetus may be carried to term, it is usually removed abdominally as soon as it is diagnosed. The placenta should be left in place unless it can be easily removed without endangering the adjacent maternal structures. Ovarian pregnancy is treated by oophorectomy. The rare cervical pregnancy usually requires hysterectomy to control hemorrhage.

Trophoblastic Growths

This group of lesions includes *hydatidiform mole, invasive mole* (chorioadenoma destruens), and *choriocarcinoma*. Hydatidiform mole, a developmental anomaly that may have hyperplastic and dysplastic trophoblast, consists of grapelike vesicles without an embryo. Many moles may arise as blighted ova. The molar villi are *edematous* and *avascular*. The mole often presents with *bleeding* in the *first half of pregnancy*, occasionally with pain, particularly if the uterine growth is rapid. In about half the cases, the *uterus* is *larger* than the dates would indicate. *Abortion* of the mole usually occurs at about *five months'* gestation or earlier, and the first indication of the disease is often the *passage of vesicles*. Severe *hyperemesis*, *preeclampsia* before the twenty-eighth week, and *anemia* are suggestive of the disorder. Since *theca lutein* cysts are present in about one third of the cases, adnexal masses may support the diagnosis. These tumors should not be excised because they regress after the trophoblastic tissue has been removed. An unusually *high titer of chorionic gonadotropin*, especially after the one-hundredth day of pregnancy, helps to confirm the diagnosis of mole. Twins and hydramnios must be excluded.

Diagnosis of mole can be made accurately by *ultrasound; amniography* and absence of fetal parts on radiologic examination are also helpful. As soon as diagnosis is made the mole should be evacuated. *Oxytocin* is used to decrease the size of the uterus; a *gentle curettage* with spongestick or suction may then be performed. Sharp curettage is permissible only after the size of the uterus is sufficiently reduced to minimize the chance of perforation. *Blood* should be available during the procedure. *Hysterotomy* is sometimes required in a uterus that does not respond to oxytocin. In older multiparas *hysterectomy* may be indicated. Because one in about five moles is followed by *choriocarcinoma* or *invasive mole*, *follow-up* by hCG *titers* and *chest films* to detect metastatic or persistent disease is mandatory. Invasive mole and choriocarcinoma are treated with great success by *chemotherapy (methotrexate* or *actinomycin D*).

Benign mole is followed by invasive mole in about 16% of cases and by choriocarcinoma in about 2.5% of cases. Since hCG titers are a mainstay of the follow-up, pregnancy should be interdicted for a year to avoid confusion with persistent trophoblastic disease. If after passage of a mole, the hCG titer is still positive a month later, persistent disease should be suspected. If the uterus is still large or if bleeding continues, the suspicion should be greater. Follow-up should be continued for one year. Chemotherapy is indicated for persistent or metastatic trophoblastic disease. Curettage is repeated and the tissue submitted for histopathologic diagnosis.

Choriocarcinoma comprises plexiform columns of trophoblast without a villous pattern. Whereas this disease was formerly almost 100% fatal, chemotherapy may now effect cures of greater than 80%.

Moles occur only about once in 2000 pregnancies in the United States but the prevalence is much greater in Hong Kong and other parts of Asia. It is relatively more common at the extremes of reproductive life. Many moles are triploid and almost all are chromosomally female. In molar pregnancy the chorionic somatomammotropin titer is relatively low. Some authorities prefer to administer methotrexate or actinomycin before evacuation of a benign mole, but many reserve these drugs for proven or suspected metastatic or persistent disease.

Invasive mole, which at first spreads locally, may penetrate the myometrium deeply and cause serious hemorrhage. Unlike choriocarcinoma it maintains a villous pattern. Both hysterectomy and chemotherapy have been effective therapy for invasive mole. Choriocarcinoma metastasizes rapidly and widely. Its presenting sign may often be referable to a metastasis in the lung, vagina, liver, or brain. Although this lesion is preceded by mole in about half the cases, it may also be preceded by abortion, term intrauterine pregnancy, or ectopic pregnancy. Pregnancies have followed the successful treatment of choriocarcinoma.

Choriocarcinomas are placed in the category of high risk when any of the following pertains: prolonged delay before treatment (four months or more), a high initial titer of hCG (100,000 IU/liter or more), or metastases to brain or liver. Such patients should receive triple therapy, which comprises methotrexate, actinomycin D, and chlorambucil. Radiotherapy and neurosurgical procedures are employed in treating cerebral metastases. Side-effects of methotrexate may be reduced by citrovorum factor rescue.

Premature Labor

The onset of labor is considered premature when it occurs *before the 36th week*, when the fetus normally weighs *less than 2500 g* (the lower limit of maturity). A fetus that weighs between *1000 and 2499* g is considered *premature*, and one between *500 and 999* g is *immature*. A fetus that is born weighing *less than 500* g (the lower limit of viability) is an *abortus*.

The basic *cause* of premature labor is *unknown* although it is often associated with *premature rupture of the membranes*. Less commonly, premature labor may be ascribed to *maternal systemic disorders* including infections, second and third trimester *uterine bleeding*, and *uterine anomalies*. Prematurity is the *leading cause of perinatal mortality and morbidity*.

Treatment of premature labor is *bedrest* and mild sedation, although attempts to stop it are generally unsuccessful and often unwise. In the management of premature labor, *narcotics* and other drugs that cross the placenta and depress the fetus should be *avoided* whenever possible. Delivery should be conducted under *regional or local anesthesia* with *episiotomy;* it should be accomplished spontaneously or by elective *outlet forceps.* The fetal prognosis depends on *maturity* and *obstetric management.* Expert *neonatal care* is a major factor in successful outcome.

About 5 to 10% of all labors are premature. Prematurity is the cause of about two thirds of all cases of perinatal mortality and morbidity. In addition, it is a major etiologic factor in cerebral palsy and mental retardation. In only a minority of cases can a cause for prematurity be found. Conditions known to be associated with prematurity include chronic vascular disease of the mother, preeclampsia-eclampsia, abruptio placentae, placenta previa, hydramnios, plural gestation, uterine malformations and tumors, and certain fetal anomalies. Maternal pyelonephritis and other infections are associated with an increase in the rate of prematurity.

Infants of mothers who smoke weigh less than those of mothers who do not, although the infants of smokers may not be premature by dates. Low socioeconomic status and poor nutrition may be conducive to prematurity. Many drugs, including alcohol and uterine relaxants, have been used in an attempt to stop labor, but their effectiveness in reducing perinatal morbidity and mortality remain to be proved by controlled clinical experiments.

EtOH?
Progesterone?
- Isoxsuprine?
→ β agonist
- Terbutaline

Premature Rupture of the Membranes

Rupture of the membranes is defined as premature when it occurs more than an hour *before the onset of labor.* The *aggressive management* of this condition depends on *delivery within 24 hours of rupture of the membranes.* If the fetus is *1800 g* or more in weight, prompt delivery is attempted. The preferred method is *oxytocin* induction if there are no contraindications to the drug. Otherwise, cesarean section is required, although this operation is rarely necessary on the basis solely of ruptured membranes. If the fetus is judged to weigh *less than 1800 g*, and the mother is *afebrile*, *expectant management* may be justified until the fetus reaches the desired weight. During this period, vaginal and rectal examinations should be avoided whenever possible. In many institutions aggressive management is carried out with fetuses estimated to weigh *1500 g* or more. Still other centers with excellent facilities for intensive neonatal care prefer to deliver babies with even lower estimated weights.

If the patient is *febrile* and the cause is judged to be *amnionitis*, *delivery* is indicated regardless of the weight of the fetus. Antibiotics are usually given after the endometrial cavity is cultured. In all cases of premature rupture of the membranes, *cultures* should be obtained from the membranes and the infant's nasopharynx. The aggressive management is not universally practiced.

Although premature rupture of the membranes may occur at any stage of pregnancy, its incidence increases as term is approached. The basic cause is unknown, but the condition is associated with premature delivery, maternal sepsis, and increased perinatal mortality and morbidity. Near term it is followed by the onset of labor within 24 hours in about 80% of cases, but the earlier in pregnancy premature rupture of the membranes occurs, the longer is the latent period (time between rupture and onset of labor.) Diagnosis of rupture of the membranes may be difficult. Nitrazine paper is often used to detect alkaline fluid, which is presumably amniotic. A "fern" pattern, fetal epithelial cells, hair, or fat globules suggest rupture of the membranes.

Placenta Previa

Placenta previa and abruptio placentae are the two most common causes of serious *third-trimester bleeding*. Placenta previa is characterized by *painless vaginal bleeding* in the third trimester. It is an important example of the principle that the *incompletely separated placenta* leads to *maternal hemorrhage*. If the fetus is judged to be under 2500 grams (*premature*) and neither subsequent bleeding nor labor ensues, *expectant management* may be attempted; that is, no attempt at delivery is made until an estimated weight of 2500 grams is attained. If severe or continuous bleeding occurs, if the patient goes into labor, or if the fetus is already mature, expectant management is inapplicable and the patient must be delivered promptly, usually by *cesarean section*.

In the most extensive variety of placenta previa (*total*), the entire internal os is covered by placenta. In the *partial* variety, only a portion of the internal os is covered. In the least extensive varieties (*marginal* placenta previa and *low-lying* placenta), the placenta barely encroaches upon the internal os.

Definitive diagnosis is made only by *digital palpation* of the placenta. This procedure must not be performed, however, except in the *operating room*, where immediate cesarean section may be accomplished if placenta previa is found. This is the *double setup* for examination and possible cesarean section. *No vaginal or rectal examinations* are permitted in a patient with suspected placenta previa except in the operating room.

Placenta previa occurs once in about 200 pregnancies. Its incidence increases with increasing maternal age and parity. It is associated with defective vascularization of the decidua and occasionally with partial placenta accreta. Abnormal presentations (transverse lie and breech) and twins are found more commonly with placenta previa. There is a tendency to repetition in subsequent pregnancies. Placenta previa must be distinguished from heavy "show." In case of doubt the patient should be hospitalized for diagnosis.

With placenta previa the uterus is of normal consistency and is nontender, unlike that of typical abruptio placentae. Placenta previa rarely occurs before the seventh month, and the first hemorrhage is rarely if ever fatal. On initial examination a speculum should be gently inserted into the vagina to rule out nonobstetric causes of vaginal bleeding such as carcinoma of the cervix or lacerations. For all bleeding patients, blood should be typed and crossmatched and an intravenous infusion should be started through a large-bore needle. If the patient is anemic, blood should be transfused.

Although diagnosis is definitively made only by digital examination, other techniques may be used: placental arteriography (transfemoral), amniography, isotopic scans of the placenta, soft-tissue x-ray, and (safest and quite accurate) sonography.

The large majority of patients are delivered by cesarean section, including all primigravidas and all patients with total and partial varieties. Vaginal delivery by simple rupture of the membranes may occasionally be indicated in a case of low-lying placenta in a multipara with minimal bleeding. Cesarean section reduces both antepartum bleeding and traumatic bleeding at delivery and post partum from injury to the friable lower segment. Less than half of all cases of placenta previa may be managed expectantly. The maternal mortality of well-managed cases should approach zero, but the perinatal mortality remains high because of prematurity and fetal hypoxia.

Abruptio Placentae

Abruptio placentae, the *premature separation* of the *normally situated placenta* after the twentieth week of gestation, is the other major cause of third-trimester bleeding. Abruption is classified as either severe or mild, depending upon the degree of separation of the placenta from the uterine wall. The bleeding may be confined to the uterus as in a *retroplacental hematoma* with no external bleeding (*concealed hemorrhage*), usually the *more serious* form of the disorder. If blood escapes into the vagina, *external* hemorrhage results.

Signs and symptoms depend on the degree and the duration of the separation. Maternal signs and symptoms may include vaginal *bleeding, shock* (if the bleeding is severe), and *uterine tenderness and rigidity*. With severe or rapid bleeding *fetal distress* or *fetal death* may occur. If only slight external bleeding occurs in the absence of uterine pain or rigidity or fetal distress, bedrest and careful observation may suffice temporarily. A *hard uterus*, usually indicating retroplacental bleeding, and fetal distress suggest severe abruption and the need for *rapid delivery*.

The route of delivery is determined by obstetric factors and the speed with which vaginal delivery may be anticipated. If there is no contraindication to *oxytocin,* it should be used together with *rupture of the membranes* when delivery through the vagina can reasonably be expected within *six to eight hours.* In all other circumstances *cesarean section* is required. Severe abruption may be complicated by maternal *hypofibrinogenemia* and *acute renal failure.*

The primary reason for rapid delivery is to *forestall* these *serious complications,* which may increase as the interval between abruption and delivery is prolonged. Aggressive management of abruption, based on the presumptive danger of time-related maternal complications, is not, however, universally practiced. Excellent results have been obtained in many institutions that do not require delivery within eight hours, as long as the maternal blood pressure and renal perfusion remain normal.

Abruptio placentae occurs in about 1% of all pregnancies. The exact frequency depends on the criteria for diagnosis. The precise cause is unknown, although a vascular lesion of the decidua frequently appears to be an underlying factor. Hypertension is associated with abruptio placentae in about one third to one half of cases, chronic hypertension more often than preeclampsia. Maternal mortality should not exceed 1% in well-managed cases, but fetal mortality depends primarily on the extent and acuteness of the separation and the degree of fetal maturity.

The first step in management involves typing and cross-matching of blood. The remaining steps include: monitoring of urinary output and possible use of mannitol as an osmotic diuretic to maintain a urinary flow of 100 ml/hr, monitoring of central venous pressure to avoid overhydration (not over 12 cm of water), administration of fibrinogen when the level falls to 100 mg%, and most important, emptying the uterus within six to eight hours by amniotomy and oxytocin or by cesarean section. The use of heparin in treating the consumptive coagulopathy that may occur in the severe forms of this disorder is controversial and potentially dangerous. Effusion of blood within the uterus in cases of severe abruption may produce a bluish discoloration (Couvelaire uterus). It is not necessary to remove the uterus except in the rare event that it fails to contract in response to oxytocin.

Trauma, short cord, and folic acid deficiency are not important etiologic factors. The earlier in pregnancy an abruption occurs, the more it resembles a late incomplete abortion.

The most trivial degrees of separation may include rupture of the marginal sinus. There is about a 10% likelihood of recurrence of abruption in subsequent pregnancies.

Other obstetric conditions in which hypofibrinogenemia occurs include amniotic fluid embolism, fetal death, and severe postpartum hemorrhage. Epsilon-aminocaproic acid is generally contraindicated unless an unequivocal excessive activator activity or hyperplasminemia can be demonstrated. Successful management of the renal failure depends on close cooperation with the "dialysis team."

Dystocia: Uterine Dysfunction

Dystocia (difficult labor), or *failure to progress in parturition,* is caused by one of three main factors or combinations of them: *abnormalities of uterine contractions* (*uterine dysfunction*); *abnormalities of size, presentation, or development of the fetus;* and *abnormalities of pelvic size* or *architecture.* Pelvic contraction is often associated with uterine dysfunction. *Together* they are the *most common* cause of dystocia.

Principles of management of all forms of dystocia include *pelvic mensuration* (manual or radiologic, if in doubt). In any dystocia the *labor* must be carefully *monitored* with respect to *uterine contractions, dilatation* of the cervix, and *station* of the presenting part. If *cephalopelvic disproportion* is discovered, a *cesarean section* must be performed and *oxytocin* stimulation is *contraindicated. Abnormalities* of the *fetal heart rate* with or without *meconium* must be detected as soon as possible. Ideally all patients are to be *monitored* to detect *fetal distress* early and to effect *prompt delivery.*

Uterine dysfunction may result from *subnormal* contractions or *abnormal contractions. Subnormal,* that is, weak or infrequent, contractions are the main indication for *oxytocin* stimulation. In *abnormal* contractions there is a *lack of fundal dominance* (gradient from top to bottom of the uterus) or *asynchrony* of uterine contractions. Uterine dysfunction is most commonly confused with *false labor,* which requires no treatment. *Primary* uterine dysfunction is present from the *onset of labor.* It is essentially a *prolongation of the latent phase. Secondary* uterine dysfunction begins *after labor* has *begun normally.* It results from an *overdistended uterus, disproportion,* premature administration of *analgesia* and *anesthesia,* and *maternal exhaustion. Prolongation* of either the first or the second stage *increases perinatal mortality. Secondary* dysfunction is usually associated with contractions that are *subnormal* in amplitude or frequency. It is often designated *hypotonic,* although the term is physiologically inaccurate. *Hypertonic* dysfunction is often *primary* and the contractions are *abnormal,* with a *reversal of gradient* or *asynchrony* of impulses from the cornua. There may possibly be emotional factors in the causation of uterine dysfunction.

True labor should not be diagnosed until the cervix has reached at least 3 cm dilatation. During an effective uterine contraction, the uterus cannot be indented. Pain is not a good indication of the effectiveness of labor. In the latent phase, effacement may occur without much cervical dilatation.

Subnormal uterine contractions complicate about 4% of all labors. Even during the height of a contraction the uterus may be indented. Fetal distress occurs late; oxytocin is specific therapy; and rest is of no value.

Hypertonic uterine dysfunction complicates about 1% of all labors. It involves mostly the latent phase and it may appear to be painful out of proportion to the stage of labor. Fetal distress occurs early. Oxytocin is probably of no value, but rest and sedation for a short period of time may be tried before resorting to cesarean section.

In the management of subnormal uterine contractions it is important to prepare a *timetable of action.* The pelvic measurements, cervical dilatation, and fetal station and position must be known precisely. A *cesarean section* is to be performed if *disproportion* is discovered. When using *oxytocin* the physician must *remain with the patient,* monitoring the fetal heart rate, uterine contractions, and maternal vital signs. An intravenous infusion of dextrose and water must be started and the solution of oxytocin (10 units/liter) run into the tubing of the first infusion. The infusion should be started slowly and increased to a maximum of 20 to 30 milliunits per minute, preferably with control by an accurate pump. Higher concentrations are unnecessary and potentially dangerous. When used for proper indications, oxytocin is effective at low concentrations and after only a short period of infusion. The *intravenous route* is the most accurate, safe, and easily controlled method of administering oxytocin. Prostaglandins also have been used successfully for stimulation of labor, but ergot alkaloids and other drugs are not recommended for this purpose.

A long latent period may be defined as 20 hours in the primigravida and 14 hours in the multigravida. The cervix normally dilates at the rate of about 1.2 cm per hour in the primigravida and 1.5 cm per hour in the multipara. A minimal pressure of 15 mm of mercury is required for an effective contraction. The pressure exerted during an average uterine contraction is about 50 mm of mercury.

Contraindications to oxytocin are absolute and relative. Absolute contraindications include fetopelvic disproportion and transverse lie. Relative contraindications include advanced age (over 35 years), high parity (greater than five), and overdistension of the uterus (as with twins and hydramnios). If doubt about the propriety of using oxytocin in a particular situation remains, it is safer to avoid using the drug.

Abnormal Presentations

Fetal causes of *dystocia* include *excessive size* or *malpresentations* of a normal-sized infant (for example, transverse lie at term in a normal pelvis). This group also includes *fetal anomalies* such as hydrocephalus, double monsters, and fetal tumors. Fetal causes of dystocia are managed by *cesarean section* as soon as the diagnosis is made.

Breech presentation, in which the *sacrum* or *one or both feet* may be the *presenting part*, occurs in 3 to 4% of all pregnancies at term. Since the *largest part* of the fetus (the head) *passes* through the pelvis *last*, the *route of delivery* (abdominal or vaginal) must be *decided early*, for there can be no trial of labor. *Complications* of breech presentation include increased incidence of *prolapse of the cord* and *increased perinatal mortality and morbidity*. *Cesarean section* is indicated in all cases of *pelvic contraction* and *oversized fetus* and often in any *elderly primigravida* (over the age of 35). In all primigravidas with a breech at term, *pelvimetry* is indicated. *Sonographic* measurement of the biparietal diameter of the fetal head is most useful. Since the breech often does not fit the pelvis well, the likelihood of *premature rupture of the membranes* is increased. A *vaginal examination* should be performed immediately after this event to *rule out prolapse of the cord*. Premature rupture of the membranes must be *managed aggressively* (p. 85) to minimize intrauterine infection and perinatal morbidity and mortality.

The most common type of breech is the frank breech (knees extended and thighs flexed on the abdomen). With full, or complete, breech, both knees and hips are flexed. In frank and full breeches the presenting part is the sacrum. In footlings, one or both hips and knees are extended. The fetal head does not have time to mold and it may be trapped by the cervix if delivery begins before full dilatation. Since the cord is inevitably compressed against the inlet by the fetal head by the time the fetal umbilicus reaches the introitus, delivery must be completed within ten minutes of this time.

Although prolapse of the cord commonly occurs with breech presentation, the accident may be associated with any factor that interferes with adaptation of the presenting part to the inlet, such as transverse lie, face presentation, plural gestation, small fetus, or contracted pelvis. Treatment of prolapse of the cord depends upon the dilatation of the cervix. With full dilatation, a forceps delivery of a vertex or a breech extraction may be performed if there are no obstetric contraindications. When the cervix is incompletely dilated and the fetus is alive, cesarean section should be performed.

The use of cesarean section for delivery of breeches has increased markedly in recent years. Certain obstetricians recommend abdominal delivery of virtually all primigravidas with breech presentations. Other indications for cesarean section include footling breeches (to prevent prolapse of the cord) and premature breeches (to prevent entrapment of the head by an incompletely dilated cervix).

Breech presentation may be associated with hydramnios, hydrocephalus, placenta previa, uterine septa, prematurity, and twinning. Since about 40% of fetuses present by the breech at the twenty-eighth week, whereas only 3 to 4% present by the breech at term, it is evident that 90% turn spontaneously during the third trimester. The perinatal mortality associated with breech presentation at term is three times that of vertex presentation.

External version (p. 128) may be attempted in the last six weeks of pregnancy without anesthesia, although reversion to breech presentation often occurs. The preferred method of delivery is partial breech extraction, or assisted breech delivery. In this procedure the breech delivers spontaneously to the umbilicus. In spontaneous breech delivery the entire fetus is born without assistance, as commonly happens with prematures. Total breech extraction is performed only for difficulties such as fetal distress or a prolonged second stage.

Oxytocin must be used with caution in any breech presentation. Complete breech extraction requires deep uterine relaxation. Fetal injuries associated with breech delivery include fractures of the clavicle, femur, humerus, and spine; injuries to the brachial plexus; hemorrhage in the adrenal, kidney, liver, and spleen; intracranial bleeding; and hypoxia leading to brain damage. The perinatal mortality and morbidity are increased by these factors as well as by prematurity, congenital anomalies, and associated maternal conditions such as placenta previa.

In transverse lie, the long axis of the fetus is perpendicular to that of the mother and the shoulder is the presenting part. This presentation occurs once in about 300 labors. Vaginal delivery of a term-sized fetus in this presentation is usually impossible and cesarean section is therefore required. Transverse lie is associated with a relaxed abdominal wall (high multiparity), pelvic contraction, placenta previa, prematurity, plural gestation, and uterine myomas.

The mother's prognosis in transverse lie is worsened because of spontaneous and traumatic (version) uterine rupture and associated conditions such as placenta previa and advanced age. The fetal prognosis is poor because of traumatic delivery, hypoxia, infection associated with premature rupture of the membranes, and prolapse of the cord. A neglected transverse lie may lead to serious intrauterine infection, which may require cesarean hysterectomy (p. 124).

With face presentations the head is completely extended and the chin is the presenting part. This presentation occurs once in about 400 labors. It should be recognized early and cephalopelvic disproportion, which is frequently associated with face presentation, excluded. A cephalic prominence on the same side as the fetal back suggests face presentation. If the chin is anterior and there is no disproportion, vaginal delivery may be expected. If the chin remains posterior at term, cesarean section is required for delivery.

Brow presentation is usually transitional from a fully extended to a fully flexed position. It persists in only 1 in 1000 to 1 in 1500 deliveries. A persistent brow with a term fetus or any cephalopelvic disproportion requires delivery by cesarean section. The perinatal mortality of brow presentation is several times that of vertex presentation.

Occiput posterior is essentially a normal positional variant often associated with anthropoid and android pelves. This position may be associated with a prolonged second stage and incomplete flexion of the head. Most occiput posteriors turn spontaneously to occiput anterior positions. Persistent occiput posteriors may be delivered by rotation (manual or forceps) to an anterior position or as occiput posteriors (face to pubis). Cesarean section should replace difficult midforceps delivery of occiput posteriors.

Pelvic Contraction

Absolute contraction of the pelvic *inlet* or *midpelvis* will *prevent vaginal delivery* of a normal-sized infant. An unusual pelvic configuration even without absolute contraction may necessitate cesarean section. When the major *diameters* of the pelvis are at or *below critical values, oxytocin* must be used with *great caution* in the presence of a normal-sized fetus. Minor degrees of pelvic contraction are often associated with *uterine dysfunction*.

The critical diameters, in centimeters, of the pelvis are as follows:

	Anteroposterior	*Transverse*
Inlet	10.0	12.0
Midplane	11.5	9.5

A contracted pelvis may result from malnutrition, injury, or congenital anomalies. Maternal complications include prolonged labor, premature rupture of the membranes, uterine rupture, and fistulas. Fetal complications include infection, prolapse of the umbilical cord, and intracranial hemorrhage.

The ideal obstetric pelvis has a roundish inlet with a broad and deep posterior segment. The lateral walls slope gently toward the symphysis to form a broad and deep forepelvis. The sacrosciatic notch is wide; the pubic arch is wide; and the bones are light. A flat, or platypelloid, pelvis favors a transverse position of the head and a long, or anthropoid, pelvis favors a posterior mechanism of labor.

Plural Gestations

Plural gestations (twins and higher multiples) occur in *more than 1%* of all pregnancies. The fetuses may lie in any combination of presentations. The prevalences of *hydramnios, preeclampsia,* maternal *anemia,* and *prematurity* are increased with plural gestation. The *second twin* should be delivered within *15 to 30 minutes* of the *first twin.* After delivery of the first infant, the uterine end of its *cord* should be *clamped. Oxytocin* and *blood* should be available in such situations to prevent or combat postpartum hemorrhage.

The rate of monovular twinning is constant in all maternal age groups and races. Dizygotic (binovular, fraternal) twins are more common in the black population. With twins the uterus is usually larger and more than the usual number of fetal small parts may be palpated. Two fetal heart beats differing by more than 10 beats per minute suggest twins. The infants in plural gestation usually deliver before term. Death of one or both twins during labor or delivery may result from operative interference, prolapse of the cord, or premature separation of the placenta.

Monochorial twinning may lead to the transfusion syndrome, with the donor twin malnourished and the recipient twin plethoric. Monoamnionic twins may have knotted cords, which may lead to death of one or both fetuses. Twins have a greater prevalence of vasa previa and velamentous insertions of the cord, which may result in injuries to the umbilical vessels and fetal hemorrhage. In vasa previa, the umbilical vessels traverse the lower uterine segment in advance of the presenting part. In cases of velamentous insertion of the cord into the fetal membranes, the umbilical vessels course between amnion and chorion unsurrounded by Wharton's jelly.

Postpartum Hemorrhage and Obstetric Injuries

Postpartum hemorrhage is defined as loss of *more than 500 ml* of blood during the *first 24 hours* after delivery. It is the most common variety of severe hemorrhage in obstetrics and a major factor in maternal mortality. The three principal causes of postpartum hemorrhage are *uterine atony, trauma* to the genital tract, and *retained secundines* (placenta and membranes). Uterine atony, the most common cause, may result from any condition that leads to *overdistension* of the uterus. Injuries result primarily from *traumatic deliveries* and inadequately repaired *episiotomies*. Retained secundines usually result in a somewhat more *delayed* hemorrhage.

Diagnosis and treatment must be performed with minimal

delay. As soon as excessive bleeding is recognized, a *large-bore needle* is inserted into a vein for administration of *fluids,* and *blood* is crossmatched and made available. In a healthy young woman the blood pressure and pulse rate may remain almost normal until a great deal of blood has been lost, at which point *shock* may suddenly develop.

Transfusion should always be instituted *before* the patient has lost *1000 ml* of blood. The first step in management is *uterine massage*. An *oxytocic* agent is administered if the uterus is hypotonic. If bleeding continues from a firmly contracted uterus, injuries to the genital tract are a more likely cause. After any difficult delivery the *vulva, vagina* (including *episiotomy* site), and *cervix* should be *inspected* and any *lacerations repaired.* The *uterus* should be manually *explored,* especially if the cervix is deeply lacerated, to rule out *injury* and to remove any *placental fragments.* The delivered placenta should be carefully examined to rule out *incomplete removal*. The blood should be observed to see whether it clots and to rule out *hypofibrinogenemia,* which is treated by intravenous administration of 4 g of fibrinogen. If the uterus is still bleeding after lacerations have been repaired and after oxytocic agents have been administered, uterine *bimanual compression* and preparation of the patient for *laparotomy* should be performed. The *uterus* should *not be packed.*

Uterine atony accounts for about 90% of all cases of immediate postpartum hemorrhage. It should be anticipated in prolonged labor, high multiparity, and general anesthesia with agents that relax the uterus. It is more common with plural gestation, hydramnios (2000 ml or more amniotic fluid), excessively large infants, and myomas. The likelihood of uterine atony is greatly reduced by the proper use of oxytocic agents. One ampul (10 units) of oxytocin may be administered intramuscularly or by intravenous drip after delivery of the infant, but not directly into the vein in a single rapid injection. Methylergonovine maleate (0.2 mg) may be given intravenously after delivery of the placenta.

Trauma to the genital tract results from tumultuous labor, difficult forceps delivery and internal podalic version, injudicious use of oxytocin before delivery, and mismanagement of the third stage (forceful attempts to remove the placenta prematurely). After any difficult labor or delivery the genital tract should be systematically inspected. If a uterine rupture is encountered or suspected the patient should be transported without delay to the operating room. Ligation of the hypogastric artery or hysterectomy may be required for hemostasis.

The delivered placenta should be carefully inspected to rule out retention of a cotyledon, as indicated by a defect in the maternal surface. A torn vessel at the edge of the placenta suggests retention of a succenturiate lobe. Retained secundines and subinvolution of the placental site usually lead to postpartum hemorrhage that is delayed (from the second day to a month after delivery). Placental fragments may then be removed by polyp forceps and the subinvoluted site curetted.

Hypofibrinogenemia is a much less common cause of postpartum hemorrhage. It is often associated with severe abruption of the placenta, retention of a dead fetus for more than a month, and amniotic fluid embolism.

Uterine rupture may occur through a scar (usually cesarean section) before and during labor or though an intact organ after difficult labor or delivery. Rupture should be suspected when the uterine contractions cease and the fetal heart tones are lost in the presence of severe abdominal pain. A classical cesarean section scar may rupture early (before the onset of labor), whereas a low-segment scar more often ruptures during labor.

Preeclampsia-Eclampsia

Preeclampsia, characterized by *hypertension, edema,* and *proteinuria, develops after the twentieth week* of gestation and appears with increasing frequency as pregnancy progresses. Hypertension and at least *one* of the other signs are required for the diagnosis. *Eclampsia* is preeclampsia with *convulsions,* which may occur ante partum, intra partum, or post partum. The cause of preeclampsia is unknown; the leading, but unproved, hypothesis attributes it to *uteroplacental ischemia.* It is predominantly a disorder of *primigravidas;* when it occurs in multiparas there usually is some predisposing factor. Preeclampsia is often confused with *essential hypertension* or *renal disease*, either latent and revealed by pregnancy, or frank but unobserved because the patient was not seen until late in gestation. A blood pressure of 140/90 or higher before the twentieth week suggests chronic hypertension antedating pregnancy. Preeclampsia may be *superimposed* on chronic hypertension. Gestational hypertension without either proteinuria or edema and with disappearance after delivery is called *transient*.

A major aim of prenatal care is to detect incipient preeclampsia early in its course, for its progression to eclampsia usually can be prevented. Although the only specific treatment is *termination of pregnancy*, early signs are treated by *bedrest and restriction of sodium*. The objectives are to *prevent convulsions* and to *salvage the infant* with minimal trauma to the mother. The blood pressure, weight, and proteinuria should decrease. If they do not and the patient is within four weeks of term, termination of pregnancy is desirable. It the patient is several weeks from term and the preeclampsia is mild, temporization may be justified. The risks of allowing the pregnancy to continue include aggravation of the preeclampsia, fetal death, and abruptio placentae. Signs and symptoms of aggravation call for delivery despite prematurity.

Antihypertensive drugs are used only if the hypertension is so severe as to be dangerous in itself, as with a diastolic pressure sustained at more than 110 mm Hg. *Hydralazine* is the drug of choice in preeclamptic hypertension. An anticonvulsant agent, preferably parenteral *magnesium sulfate*, is used in the treatment of hyperreflexia, severe preeclampsia, and eclampsia. It is used also in patients with moderately severe preeclampsia at the onset of spontaneous or induced labor. In eclampsia, oxygen should be administered after each convulsion and *digitalis* given at the onset of pulmonary edema. As soon as the patient is conscious and oriented, *labor* should be *induced* or *cesarean section* performed. Similarly, patients with severe preeclampsia should be neither oliguric nor acidotic before pregnancy is terminated. Usually the uterus is sensitive to oxytocin and labor can be induced even with an "unfavorable" cervix, but cesarean section may be preferable if vaginal delivery does not appear easy and imminent. Anticonvulsant therapy should be continued for at least 24 hours after delivery. Convulsions are associated with a significant increase in maternal mortality and perinatal loss; a major factor in perinatal loss is prematurity.

In superimposed preeclampsia, the perinatal loss is four times as great as in either preeclampsia or chronic hypertension alone. Low socioeconomic status and geographic and racial differences are alleged to be factors in the development of preeclampsia, although proof is lacking.

Hypertension is a sustained rise, over the usual levels, of 30 mm Hg in the systolic or 15 in the diastolic readings, or a sustained pressure of 140/90 or higher. "Sustained" means on at least two occasions six or more hours apart. Generalized edema, rather than pedal edema, is a diagnostic sign, although it occurs in many normal pregnant women. Proteinuria means one plus or more.

In differential diagnosis, chronic hypertension rather than preeclampsia is suggested by (1) previous hypertensive pregnancy, (2) multiparity, (3) retinal angiosclerosis, or hemorrhages and exudates, (4) cardiomegaly, (5) exorbitant hypertension, and (6) little or no proteinuria.

Factors predisposing to preeclampsia are (1) nulliparity, (2) familial history of preeclampsia-eclampsia, (3) plural gestation, (4) diabetes, (5) chronic hypertension, (6) hydatidiform mole, with which preeclampsia may occur as early as the fourteenth week, (7) fetal hydrops, and (8) extremes of age.

Inconstant signs of incipient preeclampsia are gains of three or more pounds per week, increasing edema of the hands and face, and a trend to rise in blood pressure. Occasionally the onset of preeclampsia is explosive. The presence of one or more of the following marks preeclampsia as severe: (1) sustained blood pressure of 160/110 or higher, (2) proteinuria of more than 5 g/liter, (3) urinary output of less than 400 ml/24 hrs, (4) cerebral or visual disturbances, and (5) cyanosis or pulmonary edema. Others are hyperreflexia, hemoconcentration, and epigastric pain.

Magnesium sulfate is given intravenously as an initial dose of 3 or 4 g in 10% solution, followed by either (a) continuous infusion of 1 to 2 g/hr or (b) 10 g in 50% solution by deep intramuscular injection, with later injections of 5 g doses at intervals of four hours. The initial dose is safe, but subsequent doses, or the continuous infusion, may not be unless (1) the knee jerk is active, (2) the urinary output is at least 100 ml/4 hours, and (3) the respiratory rate is 12 or more/minute. Calcium gluconate, 10 ml of 10% solution, is an antidote to magnesium toxicity and should always be available. If the urinary output falls below 20 ml/hour, mannitol is infused but not repeated unless the urinary volume rises to about 100 ml/hour. Furosemide or ethacrynic acid may be given intravenously but both are usually contraindicated, as are all diuretics.

Complications of preeclampsia and eclampsia include retardation of fetal growth, abruptio placentae, acute renal failure, hypofibrinogenemia, cerebrovascular accidents, hemolysis, disseminated intravascular coagulation, jaundice, and rarely, retinal detachment, hepatic rupture, and trauma incurred during convulsions. The major causes of death in eclampsia are cardiac failure, pulmonary edema, and cerebral hemorrhage.

Anatomic lesions in fatal cases of eclampsia are widespread arteriolitis, thrombosis of small vessels, hemorrhage, and necrosis. A characteristic but not wholly specific renal lesion is found in biopsies from preeclampsia women; the glomerular capillary endothelial cells are swollen and fibrin derivatives are deposited, accounting partially for the reduction in renal blood flow and the still greater decrease in glomerular filtration.

The fundamental derangements are an abnormally large retention of sodium and arteriolar spasm. There is no good evidence that diuretics and limitations of weight gain and sodium intake prevent preeclampsia; once preeclampsia has developed, however, restriction of sodium seems to be beneficial. The arterioles are sensitized to pressor substances, but no such agent has been identified as causing preeclamptic hypertension. Despite the generalized vasoconstriction, the total blood flows to most regions of the body are normal.

Almost the only helpful laboratory tests are serial measurements of proteinuria, which increases with severity, and of the hematocrit as an index to the hemoconcentration occurring in severe preeclampsia and eclampsia. Progressive or irreversible hemoconcentration denotes a bad prognosis. Hyperuricemia supports the diagnosis of preeclampsia. Significant increases in blood or plasma creatinine point to renal disease.

Ambulatory treatment of severe preeclampsia is unsatisfactory. A patient with minimal signs may be treated at home, but must be seen two or three times each week. Once the diagnosis seems definite, she should be in the hospital. A convulsion in a pregnant woman must be regarded as eclampsia until proved otherwise. Among conditions to be differentiated are epilepsy and lesions in the central nervous system. The edema and usually the proteinuria clear within a few days after delivery. In half the cases, the blood pressure returns to normal within 10 days, but may be unstable for as long as six months. In the other half, the pressure subsides more slowly, but unless the patient has underlying hypertension it will return to normal within a few weeks.

About one third of primigravidas with preeclampsia-eclampsia will have a recurrence of hypertension in later pregnancies, usually without more than mild increases; such women are likely to develop essential hypertension later. It is improbable that preeclampsia-eclampsia causes so-called residual hypertension.

Hemolytic Disease of the Newborn

Pregnancy may initiate *immunologic sensitization* of a mother to tissues of her fetus. The usual cause of *isoimmunization* is the *Rh factor*. In this situation an *Rh-negative mother* is sensitized by transfer of *fetal erythrocytes* to the maternal circulation, usually at the time of delivery but occasionally earlier in pregnancy. The *Rh-positive fetal cells* enter the maternal circulation through breaks in the placenta. Sensitization may also be produced by *transfusion* of Rh-positive cells into an Rh-negative mother. In both cases the maternal *anti-Rh antibodies* are transferred back to the fetus and cause hemolysis. An Rh-negative mother should have *serial titers* during pregnancy. The *antibody titers* are not good indications of the severity of erythroblastosis but rather a *screening test*. Once the *indirect Coombs' test* is positive in a titer of *higher than 1:16*, an amniotic fluid analysis (*amniocentesis*) must be done to detect the *bilirubin* levels.

In a sensitized mother obstetric management is directed toward improvement of fetal survival. The *management* and *prognosis* of the fetus are related to the *amniotic fluid analysis* and to the *histories* of *prior pregnancies*. The *unsensitized Rh-negative mother* should receive 300 μg of *anti-D* (Rh_0) *gamma globulin* (RhoGAM) intramuscularly *within 72 hours* of *late abortion* or *delivery* if her infant is *Rh-positive* or if its *blood type is unknown*. Smaller doses are adequate after early abortion. All Rh-negative mothers must have fetal cord blood tested after abortion or delivery to assess the fetus' Rh-status and the presence of sensitivity.

The first pregnancy in an Rh-negative woman who has not received a transfusion of incompatible blood usually produces an unaffected child. With each successive pregnancy with an Rh-positive fetus the prognosis becomes worse. A history of prior Rh-disease or a positive maternal antibody titer requires amniocentesis at 30 weeks to detect levels of bilirubin derivatives. An optical density graph of the amniotic fluid is prepared and the peak at 450 mμ is read.

If the graph indicates isoimmunization with hemolysis before 34 weeks, an intrauterine transfusion may be required. Later in gestation early delivery and exchange transfusion are preferable. Because of gross prematurity, intrauterine transfusion is appropriate therapy only after the twenty-fifth week. After the thirty-second week, premature delivery is safer and more appropriate. Intrauterine transfusion thus finds its greatest place between the twenty-fifth and thirty-second weeks of pregnancy.

The terms Rh-positive (DD or Dd) and Rh-negative (dd) refer essentially to the presence or absence, respectively, of the antigen D, although other isoantigens such as C and c or E and e may be involved.

Not all Rh-incompatibility results in hemolytic disease of the newborn (erythroblastosis or isoimmunization). ABO-incompatibility may protect against Rh-disease. Hemolytic disease on the basis of major blood group incompatibilities is uncommon because of the wide distribution of fetal A and B antigens, as a result of which antibodies are bound elsewhere than the erythrocytes. Type O women have anti-A and anti-B antibodies, which hemolyze A and B erythrocytes before maternal sensitization to the Rh-antigens takes place.

Intrauterine death with isoimmunization may occur with cardiac failure, edema (hydrops), and ascites. The neonate may have anemia, hyperbilirubinemia, and kernicterus. The placenta in hydropic forms of erythroblastosis is large. The fetus is not jaundiced because the placenta clears its plasma of bilirubin.

In hemolytic disease of the newborn, prompt clamping of the umbilical cord is recommended and the end is left long for possible exchange transfusions. A positive direct Coombs' test on the cord blood means an affected fetus. A hemoglobin level less than 10 g or an unconjugated bilirubin value greater than 5 mg suggests the possible need for exchange transfusion. The bilirubin level should be kept below 20 mg%.

Diabetes Mellitus

Most medical complications do not alter the course of pregnancy and are themselves not altered by pregnancy. A few major exceptions are discussed on pages 105 through 118. Perhaps the most important is diabetes mellitus. *Before* the introduction of *insulin,* diabetic patients *rarely* carried their pregnancies to term or even became *pregnant.* At present the incidence of this complication of pregnancy is 1% and rising. The disorder is often first *unmasked during pregnancy.* Because of the *normal gestational changes* in *carbohydrate metabolism* and *renal function,* the diagnosis must be made with caution. Detection of urinary sugar should be made with a *glucose-specific enzyme test* to rule out lactosuria. A *glucose tolerance test* (GTT) should be performed on all pregnant patients with a family history of diabetes, a history of large infants (over 4000 g), previous children with congenital anomalies, unexplained stillbirths, habitual abortions, or significant obesity. If the GTT is normal in early pregnancy in these patients, it should be repeated in each of the subsequent two trimesters.

Pregnancy affects the diabetes and diabetes affects the pregnancy. The effects of pregnancy on the diabetes include an *alteration in glucose tolerance.* There is *hyperinsulinemia* in normal pregnancy but a decrease in the effectiveness of insulin. The vomiting of pregnancy may initially lead to insulin shock; later, as a result of starvation, ketoacidosis may be produced.

The efforts of labor may deplete the glycogen, and the increased likelihood of infection makes the possibility of acidosis greater in pregnancy. Gestational glucosuria may also stem in part from a change in the filtered load of glucose. Since the level of insulin is higher in pregnancy and its half-life is unchanged, there must be an overproduction of insulin, which may stress the pancreas. Insulin is antagonized by *human chorionic somatomammotropin;* the effect of degradation by insulinases is much less significant. Steroid hormones may further decrease glucose tolerance.

The diabetic pregnancy is complicated by an increased incidence of *preeclampsia* (perhaps fourfold), *hydramnios, large babies, fetal death,* and *congenital anomalies.* There is also an increased incidence of maternal *urinary tract infection.* The *perinatal mortality rate is increased* to 10 to 40% in insulin-using diabetics, and there is an increase in respiratory distress syndrome (probably related largely to prematurity) and neonatal hypoglycemia, hypocalcemia, and nonhemolytic hyperbilirubinemia.

The best results in management of the pregnant diabetic are provided by an obstetrician with special knowledge of *perinatal medicine.* The most important factor is *medical control* of the disease. The second principle of management is appropriately *early delivery.* With excellent management the perinatal mortality may be reduced to 10% and the maternal mortality essentially to zero. Recent reports suggest that ideal management by an expert in maternal-fetal medicine may reduce the perinatal mortality still further.

The nonovert (preclinical, Class A) diabetic is managed obstetrically almost the same as a normal pregnant patient. Uncomplicated *Class A diabetics* are generally delivered at *term.* The *overt diabetic* is managed by an obstetrician or a medical team that is concerned with maintaining strict *control of the diabetes* and ensuring *early delivery.*

The timing of the delivery depends principally upon two factors: *fetal maturity* and *fetal well-being.* Complications to be avoided during pregnancy are infections, acetonuria, and preeclampsia. *Insulin dosage* should be regulated according to *blood* sugars with the aim of maintaining normal glucose levels.

The patient should be seen weekly throughout pregnancy.

Overt diabetics are generally delivered between the *thirty-fourth and thirty-eighth weeks,* depending on the severity of the disease. Earlier delivery is indicated in more severe diabetes and in the presence of preeclampsia, repeated ketoacidosis, hydramnios, or advancing retinopathy. Prior intrauterine deaths are another indication for earlier delivery.

Fetal distress may force early delivery despite prematurity. *Estriol* values may be helpful in detecting fetal distress after the thirty-fourth week; before that time prematurity may prevent a successful outcome of the pregnancy. *Oxytocin challenge tests* and measurements of *placental lactogen* may provide additional indices of fetal distress. Despite the often large size of the *newborn* its fragile condition requires *intensive care* in the high-risk or premature nursery. *Pregnancy* should be *discouraged* in severe diabetics. *Therapeutic abortion* is indicated for progressive renal disease, retinitis with progressive visual loss, and coronary arterial disease.

Class A diabetics have an abnormal glucose tolerance test, but no clinical signs of diabetes. Class B diabetics are those whose disease began after the age of 20 or has been present for as long as nine years with no vascular disease. Class C diabetics are those whose disease began between the ages of 10 and 19 or has been present for between 10 and 19 years with no vascular disease. Class D diabetics are those whose disease began before the age of 10 or has been present for 20 years or more, with vascular disease, calcification of the vessels of the legs, or benign retinopathy. Class E diabetics have in addition calcified pelvic vessels. Class F diabetics have nephropathy, and Class R have proliferating retinopathy. The less severe diabetics often have large babies and placentas, whereas the more severe, namely those with vascular disease, often have undergrown babies and small placentas.

The oral glucose tolerance test is more sensitive and physiological, but because of variations in absorption from the gastrointestinal tract during pregnancy the intravenous test is often more useful. During labor and delivery, because of the changing requirements for insulin, the crystalline (regular) rather than a long-acting variety should be used.

The criteria for diagnosis of diabetes in pregnancy are far

from universally accepted and they differ from those used in the nonpregnant state. Furthermore, the values obtained by measuring glucose in plasma are generally about 15% higher than those in whole blood. If the fasting plasma glucose level is less than 100 mg/100 ml in the intravenous test and if the level at two hours is not greater than the fasting level, it is unlikely that the patient has diabetes.

The K value, or the rate of utilization of glucose expressed as percent per minute, is calculated from the formula:

$K = \frac{0.693}{t_{1/2}} \times 100$, where $t_{1/2}$ is the time for the concentration of glucose to decrease 50%.

This value is lower in women with decreased carbohydrate tolerance. Use of the K value allows accurate comparisons of carbohydrate tolerance, with the use of a single number rather than a curve, at various stages of pregnancy.

The patient should be hospitalized one week before anticipated delivery in order to regulate her metabolic status and to decide the route of delivery. She should be delivered by cesarean section unless an easy induction can be anticipated. The labor should be monitored and attempts at vaginal delivery abandoned if fetal distress occurs. After delivery, the maternal insulin requirement usually drops.

The problems of the neonate, in addition to those listed on page 106, include birth injuries because of large size and traumatic delivery, and congenital anomalies. The management requires careful regulation of the infant's environmental temperature, oxygen, humidity, and blood glucose. The fetal prognosis depends on the severity of the maternal diabetes, the medical management and complications of the pregnancy, fetal maturity, and neonatal care. Maternal acidosis may lead to low IQ in the offspring. The maternal prognosis is influenced by cardiovascular complications, pulmonary emboli, and severe preeclampsia or eclampsia.

During pregnancy oral hypoglycemic agents are not advised. The sulfonylurea compounds may worsen neonatal hypoglycemia. Estrogen replacement is valueless; furthermore, the use of stilbestrol during pregnancy may lead to adenosis and, rarely, adenocarcinoma of the vagina in the offspring years later (p. 164).

Estriol measurements are valuable in the management of the pregnant diabetic only if obtained daily.

Cardiac Disease

More than 1% of all pregnant patients have cardiac disease. Of this group, *rheumatic heart disease* is by far the most common, but *congenital* heart disease is forming an increasingly large proportion. *Diagnosis* of cardiac disease in pregnancy is *complicated* by the *normal gestational changes* in the cardiovascular system. The *maximal* rise in *cardiac output* during pregnancy occurs as early as the *end of the first trimester* and is *not reduced* in the *last few weeks*. As a result, the patient may *decompensate early* and at any time *up to term*. Cardiac failure occurs most commonly at the time of maximal cardiac output.

A systolic murmur may be *functional*, but diastolic and presystolic murmurs and precordial thrusts must be considered evidence of *organic heart disease* even in pregnancy. Diagnosis of heart disease requires at least one of the following: a *diastolic, presystolic,* or *continuous murmur;* unequivocal *cardiomegaly;* a loud *harsh systolic* murmur especially with a *thrill;* and an *arrhythmia.*

Mild cardiac disease may be managed *at home* with care to correct *anemia* and prevent or combat *infection* promptly. The best results are obtained through *combined management* by a cardiologist and an obstetrician. Treatment varies according to *functional class* of the cardiac disease. In general, all cardiac patients should *avoid stress* and should have *increased rest. Preeclampsia, excessive weight gain,* and *hypertension* should be treated vigorously. A *cough, rales,* or *atrial fibrillation* should arouse suspicion of impending cardiac failure. The fibrillation should be converted promptly to normal sinus rhythm.

Management of the *labor* includes well-controlled *analgesia* and *anesthesia* (p. 62) to relieve both anxiety and pain. The *second stage* should be *shortened,* and *antibiotics* should be given to prevent *subacute bacterial endocarditis. Conduction anesthesia* is appropriate for delivery of the cardiac patient. *Outlet forceps* are indicated to shorten the second stage. Hemorrhage is especially dangerous because the cardiac patient often cannot compensate for sudden hypovolemia. *Cesarean section* must be reserved for *obstetric indications.*

The *puerperium* is also a *dangerous* period for the cardiac patient. She is therefore often kept on bedrest for *7 to 10 days* after delivery. *Tubal ligation* should be *delayed* in these patients. For cardiac patients who refuse tubal ligation or for whom it is not performed for other reasons, effective *contraception* is mandatory. The patient with severe cardiac disease should be discouraged from becoming pregnant at all.

Abortion is indicated for cardiac disease only in the *first trimester,* when it can be performed by sharp curettage or suction. Later in pregnancy abortion may be as dangerous as carrying the pregnancy to term on bedrest.

Maternal prognosis depends upon the *functional capacity* of the heart, other *complications* that increase cardiac work, the quality of *medical care,* and *psychologic* and *socioeconomic* factors, for example, the possibility of hospitalization throughout pregnancy.

The anatomic changes in pregnancy that make the diagnosis of cardiac disease more difficult include elevation of the diaphragm, deviation of the heart to the left, and apparent cardiomegaly on chest film. Pulmonic and apical systolic murmurs are often hemic, presumably caused by lower viscosity of the blood during pregnancy. Dependent edema in pregnancy is not necessarily a sign of cardiac disease.

The New York Heart Association classification of cardiac disease is as follows:

Class I—No limitation of physical activity.
Class II—Slight limitation of physical activity.
(Ordinary activity produces symptoms.)
Class III—Marked limitation of physical activity.
(Less than ordinary exercise produces symptoms.)
Class IV—Complete limitation of activity.
(Insufficiency at rest, that is, cardiac failure.)

Because decreased cardiac output leads to decreased utero-placental circulation and function, the fetuses of cardiac patients are often undergrown. Patients in Classes I and II may be managed on an ambulatory basis during the early months of pregnancy. Patients in Classes III and IV must be hospitalized throughout pregnancy. Although pregnant women in Classes I and II rarely go into failure, they must be watched carefully at frequent antepartum visits.

Warning signs include basal rales, dyspnea, tachycardia, and increasing edema. Optimal management includes bedrest for 10 hours a day, rest for half an hour after each meal, employment of household help, avoidance of contact with respiratory infections, and reporting of any so-called cold. If decompensation occurs, morphine, oxygen, digitalis, rotating tourniquets, and diuretics may be lifesaving.

During the puerperium, hemorrhage, infection, and thromboembolism, which are more serious than in normal patients, must be avoided. Class III patients ideally should not become pregnant. If they do, they must remain in bed throughout the pregnancy. Abortion for medical reasons should be performed only in the first trimester. Delivery by any route of a patient in failure carries a very high mortality.

Any infection in a woman with valvular heart disease must be treated with massive antibiotics after blood cultures are obtained. If the patient requires anticoagulants, heparin is the drug of choice because it does not cross the placenta.

Maternal hypoxia may lead to abortion, intrauterine death, and prematurity. Kyphoscoliotic heart disease may lead to cor pulmonale.

A cesarean section may be indicated in patients with coarctation of the aorta to prevent rupture of the vessel. There is probably no residual cardiac damage or shortening of life expectancy as a result of pregnancy in any patient with cardiac disease.

Rubella

Rubella (German measles) is the *most important* of the *few viral diseases* known to cause *congenital anomalies* in the human fetus. In the mother it is usually a mild disease that causes fever, headache, lymphadenopathy, and a pink, confluent macular rash. The *rash* appears one week after the *viremia*. The peak of *antibody titer* follows the rash by one or two weeks. The fetus is most severely affected when the mother's viremia coincides with the period of *organogenesis*. The *congenital rubella syndrome,* acquired transplacentally, comprises numerous fetal abnormalities, involving the eye (cataracts, microphthalmia, and chorioretinitis), heart, ear, central nervous system, and other organs. The infants may have microcephaly, deafness, major arterial defects, and low birth weight. In addition, there may be osseous and hematologic changes and mental deficiency. Infants born with the congenital rubella syndrome may *excrete* the *live virus.*

The diagnosis of maternal rubella is suspected on the basis of clinical signs and symptoms, but confirmed by a *rise in antibody titer* as demonstrated by *hemagglutination inhibition* reactions. There is *no effective therapy* for the disease, but *abortion* is often performed to prevent birth of a malformed fetus.

The susceptible female population should be identified and *vaccinated* with a strain of live rubella virus. Pregnant women, however, must not be immunized with live virus, and *pregnancy* should be *interdicted* for at least *three months* after active immunization of the mother.

The earlier in pregnancy the mother contracts rubella, the greater is the likelihood of congenital anomalies in the fetus. Viremia at four weeks' gestation is accompanied by a greater than 50% chance of fetal anomalies; by 12 weeks the likelihood has dropped to 10%. The use of gamma globulin in the mother is controversial, for the clinical signs may be masked without affecting the viremia.

If the titer in the first hemagglutination inhibition test is positive in a 1:10 or greater dilution immediately after clinical signs of the disease, the patient may be considered immune. If it is positive only at dilutions of 1:8 or less immediately after the rash and it rises fourfold or more 10 to 14 days later, the patient very likely has had a viremia even in the absence of clinical signs and symptoms.

The Cendehill strain of rubella vaccine (0.5 to 1 ml injection) is said to cause less arthralgia than do other preparations. The practice of immunizing all prepuberal girls is questionable, however, because the antibody titer may fall rapidly and fail to provide immunity against rubella throughout the childbearing period.

Pyelonephritis

Acute pyelonephritis is the *most common renal disease* in pregnancy. It is usually *bilateral*, although the *right* side seems to be affected more often than the left. The onset, which is frequently *abrupt*, is heralded by *fever*, *chills*, and *flank pain*. Since it is an *ascending infection*, it may be preceded by signs and symptoms of lower urinary tract infection, such as *dysuria*, *frequency*, and *urgency*. Diagnosis is made on the basis of *leukocytes* and *bacteria* in the *urine*. *Cultures* and *sensitivity tests* determine the choice of therapy. The commonly implicated organisms are *E. coli*, *Klebsiella*, *Proteus*, *Pseudomonas*, and other *gram-negative bacilli*.

Antibiotic therapy should be *intensive* and continuous for at least *10 days*, since persistent or recurrent pyelonephritis may lead to permanent renal damage. Therapy should not be discontinued until *two successive sterile urine cultures* are obtained. *Ampicillin* (0.5 g q.i.d.) is frequently the drug of choice. The antibiotics and other antimicrobial drugs *cross the placenta* and most of them may affect the fetus. If there is *no response* to antibiotics, a *urologic investigation*, including at least cystoscopy and a retrograde pyelogram, is indicated. An intravenous pyelogram may be indicated post partum to rule out obstructive uropathy or a urologic anomaly.

Dilation of the ureters and renal pelves and *decrease in peristalsis*, primarily as a result of the hormonal changes of pregnancy, predispose to urinary *stasis*. Introduction of bacteria into the bladder (*bacilluria*) leads to cystitis, which may progress as an ascending infection to involve the ureters and kidneys. *Routine catheterization* of the bladder in pregnant women is therefore to be *avoided*.

Bacteriuria is defined as 10^5 or more colony counts per ml of urine in a clean midstream specimen. About 6 to 7% of pregnant patients have asymptomatic bacteriuria, of whom about one quarter, or 1 to 2% of all pregnant women, subsequently develop pyelonephritis. It is now believed that pyelonephritis, but not necessarily asymptomatic bacteriuria, leads to an increase in the rate of prematurity.

Sulfonamides such as sulfisoxazole may be used on an outpatient basis for mild urinary tract infections. These drugs, by competing with bilirubin for albumin binding and conjugation by glucuronyl transferase, may cause jaundice and kernicterus in the newborn, particularly the premature.

Gentamicin and kanamycin may be ototoxic and nephrotoxic to the mother. Tetracyclines administered to the mother in the third trimester may lead to discoloration of the infant's deciduous teeth, and, rarely, may cause jaundice in the mother. Chloramphenicol may produce the "gray baby syndrome" and, rarely, bone marrow depression in the mother (p. 48). Nitrofurantoin should be used only for mild infections or for maintenance after the primary infection has been apparently eradicated by an antibiotic. In patients with a glucose-6-phosphate dehydrogenase deficiency, nitrofurantoin may cause hemolysis. Methenamine mandelate is not adequate therapy for frank pyelonephritis; furthermore, it may interfere with measurements of estriol.

■ Anemia

Anemia is a condition in which circulating *red blood cells* are *deficient in number* or in *total hemoglobin content.* It may be caused by *decreased blood formation* or *increased blood loss* or *destruction.* In the *nonpregnant* woman, anemia is defined as a hemoglobin concentration of *less than 12 g/100 ml.* Since there is normally a *decline in hemoglobin concentration* in *pregnancy* because of the relatively greater increase in plasma volume than in erythrocyte mass, *anemia in pregnancy* is defined as a hemoglobin concentration of *less than 10 g/100 ml.*

The most common cause (95 to 98%) of anemia in pregnancy is *iron deficiency*. Its incidence is much higher in *lower socio-economic* groups because of *poor diet*. Most women enter the reproductive age with *low iron reserves* because of either dietary deficiencies or blood loss from heavy menstruation or prior pregnancies. Increased requirements of pregnancy will exhaust the reserves of iron and produce anemia.

Maternal complications with severe iron-deficiency anemia include *dysphagia*, *angina pectoris*, and *congestive heart failure*. *Perinatal mortality* and *morbidity* are also *increased* significantly. Diagnosis of iron deficiency depends upon demonstration of a *low serum iron content* and a high *serum iron-binding capacity*. In all cases of anemia a *direct blood smear* should be examined morphologically. In a mild iron-deficiency anemia, erythrocytes may appear normal. In more severe cases, however, *hypochromia* and *microcytosis* are demonstrable. Treatment is aimed at increasing the circulating hemoglobin concentration and total body iron reserves. To this end *supplementary iron* is recommended for all prenatal patients.

Ferrous sulfate (300 mg) every day after breakfast is adequate in *normal pregnancy*. Ferrous sulfate (300 mg) *three times a day* after meals may be required for *anemia*. Parenteral iron in the form of iron-dextran may be given if there is an intolerance to oral iron or poor absorption. A *blood transfusion* is reserved for only the most serious or *refractory* cases. Therapy is evaluated by monitoring changes in hematocrit, hemoglobin content, structure of the erythrocytes, and reticulocyte count.

Pregnancy requires about 800 mg of iron (p. 27). Since the maximum absorbed from the diet is 1 mg a day, supplementary iron is required. The most common cause of failure to respond to oral iron therapy is negligence in taking the daily supplement. Plural gestations require larger supplements. Occult bleeding is a less common cause. Malabsorption without underlying gastrointestinal disease is rare but may be associated with the use of antacids.

Hereditary anemias (hemoglobinopathies) are associated with increased maternal and fetal morbidity and mortality. The most severe complications are found in patients with sickle cell anemia (SS disease) and SC disease. Five percent of American blacks may have the sickle cell trait (SA), but less than 1% have the true disease (SS). In patients with sickle cell disease there is an increased prevalence of urinary tract and pulmonary infections. As the anemia becomes more intense, pain crises become more common and the frequencies of abortions, stillbirths, and neonatal deaths increase.

Pregnant patients with SC or SS disease should receive supplemental folic acid (5 mg daily). The need for supplemental iron should be individualized.

The treatment of a crisis is oxygen, analgesics, and hydration. Patients may benefit from partial exchange transfusion. Optimally, necessary transfusions should be accomplished before delivery and at least a liter of whole blood should be available during delivery. Since serious complications may occur during pregnancy with these hereditary anemias, family size must be limited by either sterilization or at least effective contraception.

Megaloblastic anemia caused by folic acid deficiency is an uncommon cause of anemia in the United States but is reported to be important elsewhere. It is usually related to a dietary deficiency. Signs and symptoms may include fatigue, anorexia, nausea, vomiting, diarrhea, and glossitis. The diagnosis may be made by demonstration of a low hemoglobin, macrocytosis, hypersegmented polymorphonuclear leukocytes, and a low serum folate level. Specific therapy is oral or parenteral administration of folic acid (1 to 5 mg daily). The relation of folic acid deficiency to abruptio placentae has not been demonstrated.

Thyroid Dysfunction

The normal physiologic changes in the maternal thyroid gland during pregnancy are summarized on page 29. *Hyperthyroidism* in pregnancy is often caused by *Graves' disease,* which may be a result of autoimmune phenomena. It is often associated with *long-acting thyroid stimulator* (*LATS*), an IgG globulin, which crosses the placenta and may produce hyperthyroidism in the fetus. Signs and symptoms of hyperthyroidism include loss of weight, increased appetite, tremors, increased nervousness, and hyperreflexia. The diagnosis is supported by elevated levels of *free thyroid hormones*.

Severe hyperthyroidism during pregnancy must be treated to avoid "thyroid storm" at the time of delivery and possible fetal mortality. Therapy is difficult because antithyroid drugs such as *propylthiouracil* cross the placenta and may suppress the fetal thyroid. Optimal therapy of hyperthyroidism in pregnancy may be antithyroid medication and iodine to reduce the vascularity of the gland followed by partial thyroidectomy a few weeks later. Radioactive iodine should not be used during pregnancy.

Hypothyroidism is uncommon in pregnancy and most often results from prior operations on the thyroid or therapy with ^{131}I. Hypothyroid women may have decreased fertility and high rates of abortion and stillbirth. Diagnosis is made by failure of thyroid hormones to rise as usual in pregnancy and by elevated levels of TSH. Patients are treated with full thyroid replacement. Women who become pregnant while on thyroid hormones should receive full replacement for the duration of pregnancy, with normal levels of TSH as the therapeutic goal.

The easiest and least costly screening tests of thyroid function in pregnancy are the total T_4 (TT_4) and the T_3 resin uptake. The product of these two values is termed the free thyroxine index (T_7), which is approximately equal to free T_4 and is unchanged during pregnancy. Tests utilizing radioactive iodine are contraindicated in pregnancy. Inasmuch as the thyroid gland in pregnancy is not completely suppressed by exogenous thyroid hormone, the usefulness of thyroid suppression tests is limited.

Rheumatic Diseases

The effect of pregnancy on the rheumatic diseases is variable. The group comprises systemic lupus erythematosus, rheumatoid arthritis, scleroderma, polymyositis and dermatomyositis, Sjögren's syndrome, amyloidosis, necrotizing arthritis, rheumatic fever, relapsing polychondritis, and ankylosing spondylitis. The most important rheumatic diseases that coexist with pregnancy are systemic lupus erythematosus (SLE) and rheumatoid arthritis (RA).

Most patients with SLE have normal fertility, but there is an increased prevalence of abortion, stillbirth, prematurity, and small-for-dates babies, especially in patients with renal disease. Patients with nephritis may have an exacerbation of their disease during pregnancy, most often in the first trimester or post partum. Superimposed preeclampsia is common.

Treatment of SLE must be individualized but it generally consists of aspirin or corticosteroids. Antimalarials and immunosuppressants are not recommended during pregnancy. Patients with RA may have clinical remissions during pregnancy with postpartum exacerbations. RA generally has little effect on the pregnancy. Aspirin and corticosteroids are the mainstays of therapy. Gold salts, immunosuppressive agents, and other nonsteroidal anti-inflammatory agents are contraindicated in pregnancy.

■ Thrombophlebitis

Thrombophlebitis complicates only about one in 300 to 400 pregnancies, but is more common in the puerperium (p. 119). The patient may present with palpable, indurated tender cords in the lower extremities or vulva. Deep calf tenderness, tachycardia, and fever may also be found. Treatment of superficial thrombophlebitis includes bedrest, elevation of the legs, heat, and anti-inflammatory agents. If the disease is detected early, low-molecular-weight dextran may be employed. If the thrombophlebitis fails to improve or worsens with the aforementioned treatment, anticoagulant therapy is indicated, usually in the form of heparin for 10 days. Coumarin derivatives, which cross the placenta and may cause fetal hemorrhage, should be avoided throughout the later stages of pregnancy, particularly at the time of delivery. Inasmuch as these drugs may be teratogenic, they should be avoided in the first trimester as well. Deep thrombophlebitis of the legs or pelvis requires heparinization. Pulmonary emboli may necessitate ligation or plication of the vena cava and interruption of the ovarian veins.

Disorders of the Puerperium

Puerperal morbidity is any fever of *100.4° F* (38°C) or higher on any *two* of the *first 10 days post partum,* excluding the first 24 hours, as detected with an oral thermometer using a standard technique at least four times daily. Unless another cause is found, puerperal infection, often manifested by *chills, fever,* and *tachycardia,* is assumed to be *endometritis.* The other common causes of fever in the puerperium are *urinary tract infection, mastitis, thrombophlebitis,* and infection of an episiotomy site.

Introduction of bacteria into the genital tract by attendants is the main cause of endometritis. The most common offending organism is the anaerobic streptococcus. Other common pathogens are *Bacteroides fragilis, E. coli, beta-hemolytic streptococci,* and *staphylococci.* Streptococci that are normally nonpathogenic may invade traumatized tissues. When infection is limited to the endometrium, the main sign is foul vaginal discharge. Involvement of the myometrium and parametrium may produce signs of generalized pelvic infection. Cultures of the uterine cavity and blood are then obtained and antibiotics are started. When the infection causes a peritonitis, rebound tenderness, malaise, and anorexia generally occur.

Endometritis may lead to thrombophlebitis of the pelvic (uterine wall and broad ligament) or femoral variety. Thrombophlebitis should be suspected in any puerperal patient who does not respond to treatment of presumptive parametritis. Thrombophlebitis may first appear 7 to 10 days after delivery. Diagnosis is facilitated by detecting pain and swelling of the leg. Pulmonary emboli are occasionally the first sign of deep phlebitis. The treatment may involve dextran, anticoagulation (heparin or coumadin), and ligation of the vena cava (p. 118). Puerperal infection and its sequelae may be minimized by elimination of infections before labor, correction of anemia, prompt delivery after rupture of the membranes, aseptic technique, restriction of the number of vaginal examinations, and avoidance of trauma and blood loss during delivery.

Urinary tract infection results from trauma and catheterization superimposed on urinary stasis and bacilluria. Treatment is discussed on page 113.

Mastitis is treated by heat, antibiotics, and avoidance of suckling. Abscesses may require incision and drainage. Engorgement of the breasts without inflammation may be relieved by support and cold compresses. Analgesics may be required.

Subinvolution of the uterus may be caused by retained secundines, endometritis, or myomas. It produces prolonged lochia and occasionally delayed postpartum hemorrhage. Ergot derivatives are useful. If infection supervenes, antibiotics are administered. A curettage may be required to remove retained tissues or a subinvoluted placental site.

Mortality Statistics

The *maternal mortality* rate is the number of maternal deaths *per 100,000 live births* as a direct result of the reproductive process. According to some definitions the term includes all deaths of pregnant women from any causes, including those unrelated to pregnancy. The *rate* for *nonwhites* is *several times* that for *whites.* Although both rates are continuing to fall, the *differential* is *increasing,* primarily as a result of social and economic factors rather than genetic predisposition.

The most common causes of maternal deaths are often considered to be *hemorrhage, infection,* and *preeclampsia-eclampsia.* In many series *cardiac disease* and *anesthesia* are major causes. Deaths associated with *abortion* continue to account for significant maternal mortality, particularly where the procedure is limited by restrictive legislation.

Deaths may be related *directly* to *pregnancy* or to *coincident diseases* that are affected by pregnancy or may be caused by factors *unrelated* to pregnancy. Deaths from hemorrhage, preeclampsia-eclampsia, infections, vascular accidents, and anesthesia may be considered directly related to pregnancy. Deaths from *hemorrhage* have been reduced by blood *transfusion* and *hospital delivery.* Those from *infection* have been reduced by *asepsis, hospital delivery,* and *antibiotics;* and those from *preeclampsia-eclampsia* have been reduced by *prenatal care* and *early delivery* in the hospital. *Embolism* involving amniotic fluid, air, and thrombi may be considered direct results of the reproductive process. Coincident conditions that may be exacerbated by pregnancy include cardiac disease, diabetes, and anemia. Important causes unrelated to pregnancy include infections and malignant diseases, suicide, and accidents.

Perinatal mortality is the *sum* of *stillbirths* (*fetal deaths*) and *neonatal deaths* (*deaths of liveborn infants in the first 28 days of life*). A *stillbirth* is defined as an infant with *no heartbeat* who *neither breathes nor cries nor* shows any other signs of *movement.* The *fetal death rate* is the number of *fetal deaths* (deaths of fetuses weighing *500* g *or more*) *per 1000 births* (*live births plus stillbirths*). (Five hundred grams generally corresponds to *20 weeks' gestation.*) The *neonatal death rate* and the *infant mortality rate* (*deaths under one year* of age) are also calculated *per 1000 live births.*

Perinatal deaths are divided almost *equally* between *stillbirths* and *neonatal deaths.* Many *stillbirths* are caused by *maternal diseases* such as diabetes, but in a larger percentage of cases there is *no obvious cause.* The *most common* cause of *neonatal death* is *prematurity.* Othere causes of perinatal mortality include congenital malformations, obstetric trauma, intrauterine hypoxia, infection, hematologic disorders (including erythroblastosis), pulmonary dysfunction (atelectasis and respiratory distress syndrome), and iatrogenic causes. In many cases there is no sufficient pathologic diagnosis.

Between 1967 and 1974 the total perinatal mortality rate in the United States fell from 32 per 1000 to about 20 per 1000. The neonatal mortality during this period fell from 16.5 to 12.2 per 1000 live births. A goal of the American College of Obstetricians and Gynecologists is to reduce the perinatal mortality rate to 10 per 1000 by 1985. Maternal deaths per 100,000 live births fell from 83.3 in 1950 to 20.8 in 1974. Only 462 direct maternal deaths were reported in 1974, or one in 6900 births. University hospitals and referral centers may have higher mortality rates because of the greater number of high-risk patients. Many northern European countries have lower perinatal death rates, which reflect their more stable populations and general lack of poverty, and possible differences in reporting.

One factor in perinatal mortality, congenital malformations, may be genetically or environmentally induced. Intrauterine hypoxia may result from abruptio placentae; placenta previa;

prolapse, knots, or entanglement of the cord; maternal hypotension; anesthesia and analgesia; shoulder dystocia; delayed delivery of the aftercoming head; and prolonged labor.

Infections may be intrauterine or extrauterine and are usually of viral or bacterial origin. Most neonatal viral infections are acquired when the infant passes through the birth canal. Important iatrogenic causes of perinatal mortality include premature delivery and destructive operations. Maternal diseases associated with increased perinatal loss include hypertensive disorders, glomerulonephritis, urinary tract infection, diabetes mellitus, and symptomatic cardiac disease.

UNIT IV

Obstetric and Gynecologic Procedures

Cesarean Section

Delivery of a fetus through incisions in the abdomen and uterus is called cesarean section. The essence of the operation is the *hysterotomy*. As a result of improvement in surgical technique, antisepsis, blood replacement, and anesthesia, cesarean section has become a safe operation that is replacing difficult vaginal deliveries. The two main types of cesarean section are the *classical*, which involves incision of the upper contractile portion of the uterus, and the *low-segment* operation, which involves incision of the lower uterine segment after dissection of the vesicouterine peritoneum. The low-segment, or low-flap, incision is usually *transverse* although it may be vertical. Cesarean section may be combined with *hysterectomy* when it is desirable to remove the uterus for disease or sterilization.

In the United States today about *half* of all cesarean sections are *primary* and *half* are operations that are *repeated* because of a *uterine scar*. *Indications* for primary cesarean section may be *fetal* or *maternal*. A major factor in the *perinatal mortality* associated with cesarean section is *prematurity*. Ascertaining *fetal maturity* (p. 43) before elective or repeated cesarean section will minimize this threat.

Most cesarean operations in the United States are low-flap procedures. The indications for classical section are resricted mainly to certain cases of anterior placenta previa and transverse lies. Disadvantages of a classical section include greater likelihood of rupture, especially before the onset of labor, in subsequent pregnancies and a greater incidence of infection, bleeding, and adhesions. Cesarean section-hysterectomy may be indicated for neglected transverse lie with an infected uterus, myomas, carcinoma in situ of the cervix, sterilization, and postpartum hemorrhage with atony. Within the last few years several clinics in this country have revived extraperitoneal cesarean section as a means of treating actual or potential intrauterine infection.

The largest numbers of primary cesarean sections are performed for dystocia related to pelvic contraction or a large fetus. Other important maternal indications include abnormal presentations, uterine dysfunction, placenta previa, abruptio placentae, preeclampsia, hypertension, erythroblastosis, diabetes, prior vaginal plastic surgical procedures, and possibly the elderly primigravida (over the age of 35). Fetal indications include prolapsed cord and fetal distress. Fetal monitoring has provided a more logical basis for selection of cesarean section for fetal indications.

The frequency of cesarean section in the United States has risen markedly during the last few years to an average of about 11%, with many services reporting a rate of over 15%, depending on the proportion of complications in the obstetric population and the local medical attitudes toward repeating all cesarean sections. Complications of the procedure include hemorrhage (the average blood loss during cesarean section is between 800 and 1000 ml), infection, anesthetic accidents, and separation of the uterine wound. Maternal mortality of the procedure has been reduced to a minimum of 0.1%. It is related largely to the indication for the operation, the presence of infection, the duration of labor, and anesthesia. Abdominal delivery *per se*, nevertheless, involves a distinctly greater risk of maternal mortality and morbidity than does vaginal delivery. Each decision to perform a primary cesarean section must therefore be made with this increased risk in mind. Perinatal mortality is related to the indication for the operation and, in the case of repeated cesarean sections, to the prevalence of prematurity.

In about 2% of cases, a cesarean section scar will rupture in a subsequent pregnancy and about 5% of women whose uteri rupture will die—a mortality of 0.1%. If, however, 1000 consecutive cesarean sections are performed, one patient will die as a result of the procedure—again a mortality of 0.1%. Whether to repeat all cesarean sections is still a moot point, although there is general agreement that all cesarean sections performed for repetitive indications (contracted pelvis, for example) should be repeated.

Forceps

The obstetric forceps is an instrument used primarily for *traction* and *rotation* of the fetal head. Each pair of forceps consists of two branches. Each branch contains a *handle*, a *shank*, a *lock*, and a *blade*. The blade, which may be solid or fenestrated, has two curves. The *cephalic curve* corresponds to the fetal head, and the *pelvic curve* corresponds to the pelvic axis. All forceps applications must be cephalic, that is, according to the position of the fetal head.

The forceps may be applied for *fetal* or *maternal indications* or *electively*. Forceps applications are classified as *low* (*outlet*), *mid*, or *high*. A low forceps operation is performed on a vertex that is on the *perineum* with the sagittal suture occupying the anteroposterior diameter of the pelvic outlet. Low forceps may be elective (prophylactic) or indicated. A *midforceps* operation refers to an application to a head that has already engaged but has not yet met the criteria for low forceps. A high forceps operation is performed on an unengaged head. It has no place in modern obstetrics because of its potential dangers to mother and fetus.

At least 25% of deliveries in this country entail the use of forceps. The prerequisites to the application of forceps include the following: fully dilated cervix, engaged head, exact knowledge of the position and station, absence of disproportion, ruptured membranes, proper positioning of the patient on the table, appropriate anesthesia, and preferably, empty bladder and rectum. Application of forceps is usually accompanied by an episiotomy.

Maternal indications include a prolonged second stage (greater than two hours), cardiac disease (to shorten the second stage), acute emergencies such as pulmonary edema and abruptio placentae, and anesthesia that prevents voluntary expulsive efforts in the second stage. Fetal indications include prematurity (to prevent trauma to the fetal head on the perineum) and fetal distress (a heart rate lower than 100 or higher than 160 per minute between contractions, irregularity of the fetal heart, or passage of meconium).

Episiotomy

Episiotomy may be midline, or median (from fourchette into midline of perineum) or mediolateral, which involves an incision from the fourchette into the perineum at about 45 degrees from the midline. The operation is usually recommended in first deliveries and in subsequent deliveries after repair of a prior episiotomy. The operation is performed to prevent lacerations of maternal tissues and injury to the fetal head. It is generally used with forceps deliveries. Complications of inadequate repair include hematomas, urinary retention, and shock.

First-degree obstetric lacerations involve only the vaginal mucosa or perineal skin. Second-degree lacerations involve the underlying muscle and connective tissue but not the sphincter ani. A third-degree laceration involves the anal sphincter in addition. When the rectal mucosa is torn as well, a fourth-degree, or complete, laceration results.

Median episiotomy entails less blood loss, is easier to repair, and is more comfortable for the patient. It may be used in most spontaneous or low forceps deliveries in any patient with an adequate perineum. The main advantage of a mediolateral episiotomy is the decreased likelihood of its extension into the sphincter ani or rectum. Mediolateral episiotomy is logical in difficult deliveries, such as breech extraction, midforceps procedures, and very large infants. If an extension of the episiotomy occurs, the injury should be repaired immediately by an experienced obstetrician.

Induction of Labor

Labor may be induced medically (by oxytocin) or surgically (amniotomy, or rupture of the membranes). Medical induction is accomplished by means of an infusion containing 10 units of oxytocin/1000 ml of 5% dextrose in water, administered at the same rate and with the same precautions as those used for stimulation of labor (p. 91). The hazards of induction with oxytocin include rupture of the uterus, premature separation of the placenta, and fetal hypoxia. Additional complications include prematurity, uterine infection, and prolapse of the umbilical cord. Several clinics have found prostaglandins to be suitable alternatives to oxytocin for medical induction of labor.

A few of the important indications for induction are erythroblastosis fetalis, diabetes mellitus, preeclampsia-eclampsia, and premature rupture of the membranes. Induction of labor in a multipara who lives some distance from the hospital and has a history of rapid labors may be considered obstetrically indicated. When induction of labor is medically indicated, delivery should usually be accomplished within 48 hours after initiation of attempts at induction and within 24 hours after rupture of the membranes.

Strictly elective inductions may appear convenient for the patient and the obstetrician, but their advisability as a routine procedure is at best questionable. Induction is most likely to succeed if rupture of the membranes is accompanied by simultaneous initiation of an infusion of oxytocin. Success of induction is further increased when the cervix is effaced, at least 2 cm dilated, and anterior, and the fetus is mature. An unengaged head is not an absolute contraindication to amniotomy, but a double set-up should be available to cope with the possibility of prolapse of the umbilical cord.

Version

Version is manual turning of the fetus by the obstetrician from one presentation to another. Cephalic version is turning of the breech or transverse to a head, or a cephalic, presentation. This procedure is done externally without anesthesia before the onset of labor. The fetus often reverts to its original position after the maneuver. Podalic version is turning of a cephalic or transverse presentation to a breech. It is performed internally during the second stage of labor under deep general anesthesia. It is the most common cause of traumatic rupture of the uterus and has been supplanted largely by cesarean section in the United States. It is occasionally performed for delivery of a second twin but the indications for internal version of a singleton are few.

Gynecologic Procedures

Papanicolaou smear. Because *cytologic examination* of the *cervix* should *routinely* accompany physical examination of the adult woman, the method of obtaining the smear was described under physical examination (p. 16).

The smear may be interpreted as *negative, suspicious,* or *positive* for malignant cells. Another popular classification divides the smears into *five classes:* Class I, or negative; Class II, or atypical but benign; Class III, or atypical and suspicious; and Classes IV and V, or positive for malignant cells, with Class V the more distinctly malignant.

Schiller test. In this test the *squamous epithelia* of cervix and vagina are painted with a solution of *iodine* and *potassium iodide. Abnormal* epithelia of various kinds including cancer do *not take* the *mahogany* stain because they contain *little* or *no glycogen.* This test is not diagnostic of a malignant lesion, but may help to direct the biopsy to a particular site.

The toluidine blue test helps to identify abnormal areas of squamous epithelium. After painting the suspicious areas with 1% toluidine blue, the area is allowed to dry and is sponged with a 1% solution of acetic acid. The normal epithelium is decolorized. The abnormal areas, which retain the deep blue stain, may then be subjected to biopsy.

Punch biopsy. This procedure involves the removal of *single* or *multiple* pieces of tissue for histologic examination. In gynecology it is performed mainly for lesions of the *cervix* and may be included in the investigation of irregular uterine or postmenopausal bleeding. This procedure does *not* ordinarily require *anesthesia* and is generally performed in the *office.*

Colposcopy. This is a technique for examination of the cervix at a magnification of 10 to 40 times. The procedure discloses epithelial abnormalities and suggests areas for directed biopsies. Colposcopy may be used as a means of improving the rate of detection of cervical cancer in conjunction with exfoliative cytology. Satisfactory colposcopy requires visualization of the *entire squamocolumnar junction.* Colpomicroscopy is another means of direct visualization of the cervix using higher magnifications of 200 to 300 times.

Four-quadrant cervical punch biopsy has been supplanted largely by colposcopically directed biopsy. It involves biopsy of the cervix at the 3, 6, 9, and 12 o'clock positions around the external os. The squamocolumnar junction should be included in as many specimens as possible. Biopsy at the 6 o'clock position is often performed first to avoid contamination of the operative field by bleeding from above.

Cone biopsy. This is an *excision* of a *cone* of *cervical tissue* for histologic diagnosis. It is required to *rule out invasive carcinoma* when the Papanicolaou smear is positive and colposcopy has not been performed or has been unsatisfactory. This procedure is done in the *hospital.* The *base* of the cone surrounds the *external os* and the *apex* is at or near the *internal os.* The cone thus *includes* essentially all of the *endocervical canal.*

Dilatation and curettage. A *therapeutic curettage,* as performed for *incomplete abortion,* serves as both diagnosis and treatment of the condition. A *diagnostic curettage* is performed to identify a lesion in the endocervix or endometrium. It is best performed *fractionally; that is, endocervix and endometrium* are curetted in sequence and the specimens placed in separate containers for orientation and identification of the site of the lesion. For ordinary diagnostic curettage the cervical canal is scraped with a small curette before it is dilated. The *size* and *configuration* of the *uterine cavity* are first ascertained by *sounding* before the curettage. The endometrium is systematically curetted and *polyp forceps* are inserted to ensure that large lesions such as polyps have not been missed by the sharp curette.

Complications of dilatation and curettage include *cervical laceration and uterine perforation.* Curettage should therefore be done in a *hospital,* where accidents may be promptly treated. The procedure is *always indicated* for diagnosis of irregular uterine bleeding except in very *young girls. Contraindications* include *intrauterine pregnancy* and *acute pelvic inflammatory disease. Suction curettage* is the removal of the uterine contents by means of a hollow curette attached to a strong vacuum pump.

Endometrial biopsy. This procedure involves removal of a small fragment of endometrium by means of a *small sharp curette* (Novak suction curette). It is usually performed as part of the investigation of *infertility* to ascertain *ovulation* or adequacy of the *luteal phase* of the endometrial cycle. This procedure may not be adequate for the detection of *endometrial carcinoma* or atypias.

Culdoscopy. This form of *endoscopy* is the visual examination of the female pelvic viscera through the *posterior vaginal fornix.* It is used most often in the investigation of *infertility* and *endocrine problems.* It is best performed in the *hospital* but does *not* necessarily require general or regional *anesthesia.* This technique is being supplanted for many purposes by laparoscopy. *Contraindications to culdoscopy are fixed cul-de-sac and adherent uterine retroversion.*

Laparoscopy. This is an *endoscopic* procedure performed by introduction of a *telescope* through a *stab incision* in the *abdominal wall* after creation of a *pneumoperitoneum.* The laparoscope is used for a variety of *diagnostic* procedures such as the detection of tubal patency, the visualization of adnexa in cases of infertility and endocrine syndromes, and the elucidation of obscure pelvic pain. In addition, it serves many *therapeutic* purposes such as *tubal interruption.* Current improvements in the instrument are extending the range of its possible diagnostic and therapeutic uses and increasing its safety.

Culdocentesis. This procedure is the *aspiration of fluid* from the *rectouterine pouch* by *puncture* of the *posterior vaginal fornix.* It may be used to identify peritoneal fluid, blood, or pus. It is performed in certain cases of *suspected intraabdominal hemorrhage* and *abscess in the cul-de-sac.*

Colpotomy. This is an *incision* of the *posterior vaginal fornix* into the *rectouterine pouch* to *visualize* pelvic structures, perform *surgical procedures* on the adnexa, and *drain pelvic abscesses.*

Rubin test. This is an office procedure for the investigation of *tubal patency. Carbon dioxide* is introduced into the cervix through a cannula with an airtight seal. The *pressure* is *monitored* with an attached manometer. If the tubes are *patent,* a *rush of air* is heard by means of a stethoscope over the abdomen when a pressure of between 60 and 90 mm Hg is reached. At that time the pressure in the manometer drops. *Shoulder pain* usually indicates gas under the diaphragm, which provides another indication of tubal patency.

Hysterosalpingography. This is a *radiologic* procedure for investigation of *tubal patency* and visualization of *congenital anomalies* and *deformities* of the *uterine cavity* and *tube.* The radiologically visualized defects may be caused by space-occupying lesions such as polyps and myomas or extrinsic pressure. This examination can be monitored under *fluoroscopy.*

Cauterization is the induction of cellular necrosis by means of physical or chemical agents. In gynecology it is usually performed upon the cervix.

Cryosurgery is the technique of freezing by means of special probes cooled with either liquid nitrogen, Freon gas, or carbon dioxide. It is most often employed in gynecology for the treatment of benign lesions of the cervix.

Ultrasound is used more in obstetrics than in gynecology. Early in pregnancy it may be used to detect a gestational sac in the uterus or tube. Later in pregnancy it is used to measure various fetal diameters and to locate the placenta. In gynecology it may be employed to distinguish between solid and cystic tumors and between free and encapsulated fluid and to diagnose a hydatidiform mole (p. 83).

Total hysterectomy is removal of the *entire corpus* and *cervix* uteri. It may be performed through the abdominal route (*abdominal hysterectomy*) or through the vagina (*vaginal hysterectomy*).

Supravaginal hysterectomy, performed through a *laparotomy* incision, leaves the vaginal portion of the cervix. It is almost synonymous with *supracervical hysterectomy,* which leaves the entire cervix, or with *partial, incomplete,* or *subtotal hysterectomy.* None of these procedures implies removal of the tubes and ovaries, as in complete hysterectomy with *bilateral salpingo-oophorectomy. Subtotal hysterectomy* is performed today only in *emergencies* or special circumstances in which *continuation* of the operation would pose a serious *hazard* to the patient. The *total hysterectomy* is preferred because it *eliminates* the risk of subsequent *cervical carcinoma* and distressing *leukorrhea.*

Abdominal hysterectomy is generally preferred for large myomas, ovarian tumors, endometriosis, pelvic inflammatory disease, endometrial cancer, and some cases of carcinoma in situ of the cervix.

Vaginal hysterectomy is indicated for various degrees of uterine prolapse and other forms of pelvic relaxation (often in conjunction with anterior colporrhaphy or operations for the vaginal correction of stress incontinence), small mobile uteri that are bleeding, and certain small myomas. Several conditions may be treated satisfactorily by either vaginal or abdominal hysterectomy.

A major *complication* of hysterectomy is *hemorrhage,* immediate or delayed. Formation of a *hematoma* is manifested by a fall in hematocrit, a rise in temperature, and a palpable mass in the cul-de-sac or parametria. *Urinary tract* complications of hysterectomy include *pyelonephritis,* urinary tract *fistulas,* and urinary *retention. Bowel* complications include paralytic *ileus, mechanical obstruction,* and *rectovaginal fistula.* Other serious complications are atelectasis and pneumonia, local infection, evisceration, and pulmonary embolism.

Radical hysterectomy includes removal of the uterus, upper vagina, and parametria, with mobilization of the ureters. The radical hysterectomy, when performed for invasive carcinoma of the cervix (its principal indication), is usually combined with pelvic lymphadenectomy, which removes en bloc bilaterally the iliac, hypogastric, obturator, and periaortic lymph nodes.

Exenteration is the complete surgical removal of the pelvic viscera including rectum, or bladder, or both, together with all the structures removed during radical hysterectomy and pelvic lymphadenectomy. Its primary indication is persistent or recurrent cervical carcinoma. Anterior exenteration is complete surgical removal of the pelvic viscera anterior to the rectum, including pelvic lymphadenectomy, with urinary diversion. Posterior exenteration is complete removal of the pelvic viscera posterior to the bladder and urethra, including pelvic lymphadenectomy and colostomy. Total pelvic exenteration is complete removal of the pelvic viscera with ureterointestinal anastomosis and colostomy.

Simple vulvectomy, performed for benign disease, is the superficial removal of vulvar structures including skin, mucosa, and superficial fat and connective tissue.

Radical vulvectomy, performed for cancer, is the wide removal of all structures of the vulva together with adjacent skin, a portion of the mons, and subcutaneous fat down to the deep fascia and muscles. It is usually accompanied by regional lymph node dissection through single or separate incisions.

Ovarian wedge resection is the surgical removal of a longitudinal wedge of ovarian cortex and stroma extending to the hilum. It is less commonly performed today. Its principal indication is treatment of the polycystic ovary syndrome (p. 211).

Anterior colporrhaphy is the repair of a cystocele, or relaxation of the anterior wall of the vagina.

Posterior colporrhaphy is the repair of a rectocele, or relaxation of the posterior wall of the vagina.

Kelly plication is usually accompanied by anterior colporrhaphy. It is a plication of the connective tissue around the bladder neck and urethra for the relief of urinary stress incontinence.

The Marshall-Marchetti procedure is a retropubic suspension of the bladder neck for stress incontinence, performed through the space of Retzius. Sutures attach the periurethral tissue to the posterior surface of the pubic symphysis.

The Manchester operation is a vaginal procedure to correct uterine prolapse. It entails elevation of the uterus by approximation of the cardinal ligaments anterior to the cervix and is generally accompanied by cervical amputation and anterior colporrhaphy. It has been largely replaced by vaginal hysterectomy in this country.

UNIT V

General Gynecology

Gynecologic Infections

Infections of the *breast,* except those related to *pregnancy* and *lactation,* are not customarily treated by gynecologists in most parts of this country. *Postpartum mastitis* is a *pyogenic cellulitis* usually caused by *staphylococci* or *streptococci.* The mainstay of treatment is the appropriate *antibiotic,* as determined by culture and sensitivity tests. Analgesics and heat provide symptomatic relief. Treatment of an *abscess* is best accomplished by *incision and drainage.*

The *vulva* is subject to the same diseases that affect the skin of other parts of the body. *Vulvitis* often causes *pruritus,* which leads to *scratching* and secondary *trauma.* Vulvitis may cause *secondary vaginitis;* the inflammation is then designated a *vulvovaginitis.*

General dermatologic conditions that may affect the vulva include eczema, herpes, and psoriasis. Vulvar eczema is treated by removal of the irritant, steroid creams, and antihistaminics. The vulva is subject to intertrigo because of the moisture of the labia and inguinal areas. Seborrhea and folliculitis may also involve the vulva. Infestations include pubic pediculosis (phthiriasis pubis, or "crabs"), which may be treated by hexachlorocyclohexane (Kwell ointment); fleas (pulicosis); bed bugs (cimicosis); and scabies.

The primary lesions of *venereal diseases* are often found on the vulva. The *primary* lesion of *syphilis* is a painless *chancre,* which appears *three to four weeks* after exposure. The *ulcer* has *indurated* edges with a depressed center. There is edema of the surrounding skin and inguinal adenitis. The initial lesion regresses in about a month. *Darkfield* examination of the serous exudate from a chancre reveals the *spirochete.* The *serologic* test for syphilis is usually not positive until *several weeks* after the appearance of the primary lesion. Serologic tests for syphilis (STS) include the *VDRL,* which may be falsely positive in several systemic disorders.

Greater specificity may be obtained by use of the *fluorescent treponemal antibody absorption* (FTAA) test or the *Treponema pallidum immobilization* (TPI) test. The *secondary* lesions of syphilis include *condylomata lata* and *mucous patches*. The condyloma latum is a slightly raised, flat, ovoid structure that appears in clusters. It must be distinguished from condyloma acuminatum (see p. 139). Condyloma latum produces an exudate, the darkfield examination of which is positive, as are serologic tests for syphilis at this stage. The *tertiary* lesion, or *gumma,* is an uncommon finding today. The treatment of choice for primary syphilis is 2.4 million units of *benzathine penicillin* in a single intramuscular injection.

Whereas the treatment of choice for early syphilis (primary, secondary, or latent syphilis of less than one year's duration) is benzathine penicillin G because it provides effective treatment in a single visit, the Center for Disease Control recommends as an alternative treatment aqueous procaine penicillin G, 4.8 million units total, administered in a dose of 600,000 units by intramuscular injection daily for 8 days.

For patients who are allergic to penicillin, tetracycline hydrochloride (500 mg four times a day by mouth for 15 days) or erythromycin stearate, ethylsuccinate, or base, 500 mg four times a day by mouth for 15 days) may be used. These antibiotics appear to be effective but have been evaluated less extensively than has penicillin.

All pregnant women should have a *nontreponemal serologic test* for syphilis, such as the VDRL or RPR test, at the time of the first prenatal visit. The treponemal tests such as the FTA-ABS should not be used for routine screening. In women suspected of being at high risk for syphilis, a second nontreponemal test should be performed during the third trimester. Seroreactive patients should be evaluated promptly, by history and physical examination as well as by a quantitative nontreponemal test and a confirmatory treponemal test. Both of these tests should be repeated within four weeks. If there is clinical or serologic evidence of syphilis, the patient should be treated. Patients for whom there is documentation of adequate treatment for syphilis need not be retreated unless there is clinical or serologic evidence of reinfection, such as darkfield-positive lesions or a fourfold rise in titer of a quantitative nontreponemal test.

Patients at all stages of pregnancy who are not allergic to penicillin should be treated with the same doses of the drug as are used for nonpregnant patients. For patients who are allergic to penicillin, erythromycin (stearate, ethylsuccinate, or base) should be used in the doses recommended for nonpregnant patients. Although these dosages of erythromycin appear safe for mother and fetus, their efficacies are not proven. Erythromycin estolate and tetracycline are not recommended for syphilitic infections in pregnant women because of potential adverse effects on mother and fetus.

Congenital syphilis may occur if the mother has syphilis during pregnancy. If the mother has received adequate penicillin during pregnancy, the risk to the infant is minimal, but all infants should be examined carefully at birth and at frequent intervals thereafter until nontreponemal serologic tests are negative. Infants should be treated at birth if maternal treatment was inadequate or unknown or with drugs other than penicillin, or if adequate follow-up of the infant cannot be ensured.

Chancroid produces a lesion known as a soft chancre, which unlike the hard chancre of syphilis is very painful. The causative organism is the *Hemophilus ducreyi*, a gram-negative coccobacillus, which may be found in a smear or scraping of the primary lesion. A pustule appears 3 to 10 days after exposure. The primary lesion is a progressive ulcer of the vulva. Because it is difficult to culture this organism, material from the lesion must be placed in a sterile tube containing the patient's own blood and sent to the laboratory without delay. Treatment is tetracycline or a sulfa drug for 14 days.

Lymphogranuloma venereum (lymphopathia venereum, or LGV) is a venereal disease caused by one of several strains of *Chlamydia*, which are obligate, intracellular bacteria. The short incubation period of the infection results in a lesion one to three weeks after exposure. The primary infection is accompanied by fever and malaise. A suppurative inguinal adenitis (a bubo that may drain) appears two to three weeks later. Vulvar edema may progress to elephantiasis.

Complications include draining sinuses and pseudoepitheliomatous hyperplasia of the affected skin. The lymphatics of the genital, inguinal, and anal areas are involved, and rectal strictures may form. The Frei test becomes positive two to six weeks after the initial lesion and may remain positive for life. Because the complement fixation test has greater sensitivity, it has replaced the Frei test. Treatment is tetracycline or a sulfa drug for three to four weeks. Since squamous cell carcinoma may complicate this lesion, biopsy should be performed before treatment is initiated. Strictures of the large bowel may require colostomy.

Granuloma inguinale (donovanosis) is a tropical disease that affects the black population. The primary lesion is a papule, which may undergo extensive ulceration and necrosis. Unlike lymphogranuloma venereum this disease produces little lymphadenopathy, because spread occurs by the cutaneous rather than the lymphatic route. The pathognomonic finding is the Donovan body, an inclusion in the mononuclear cells. *Calymmatobacterium granulomatis,* the etiologic agent, is a heavily encapsulated, gram-negative organism. Treatment is generally tetracycline. Biopsy may be required to rule out carcinoma.

Condyloma acuminatum appears in the form of multiple papillary warty growths on the vulva, vagina, perineum, and occasionally cervix. It is caused by a *virus* and is sometimes called a venereal wart. It produces a profuse irritating *vaginal discharge,* often associated with *Trichomonas vaginalis.* Unlike the condyloma latum, this lesion has a *narrow base.* The diagnosis is made by *biopsy. Darkfield* examination for spirochetes and *culture* for the gonococcus should be done at the same time. The small lesions may be treated by the application of 20% *podophyllin* in tincture of benzoin. Care must be taken to protect the surrounding skin with mineral oil. Lesions of moderate size may be treated by cautery or cryosurgical techniques. Larger condylomas require surgical excision.

Herpesvirus hominis (*Herpes genitalis,* or *H. progenitalis*) causes vulvovaginitis. The organism may be found in smegma and the infection is *venereally* transmitted. The isolates are Type II in 90% of cases and Type I in 10%. In addition to the vulvitis and vaginitis, the infection produces a cervicitis in 75% of cases. The primary lesion is a group of *vesicles* with surrounding erythema and edema.

Herpetic infection is usually self-limited but it has been implicated in the genesis of cervical dysplasia and carcinoma (p. 167). There is no specific therapy and topical antiviral agents are ineffective. The differential diagnosis includes herpes zoster and erythema multiforme.

Gonorrhea is second only to the common cold as the most *prevalent* infectious disease in the United States. Acute gonorrhea may represent an *initial* infection or an *exacerbation* of a chronic infection. The signs and symptoms in the woman occur *three to five days* after exposure, but the primary infection may go unnoticed, rendering her an asymptomatic *carrier*. The gonococcus causes a purulent, malodorous discharge from the *urethra, Skene's glands, cervix,* and *anus*. All of these sites and the *throat* should be cultured in the attempt to make the diagnosis.

The infection is suspected when the gram-negative intracellular *diplococci* are demonstrated on *smear* and confirmed on *culture*. *Thayer-Martin* agar plates are often used for culture of gonococci. The treatment of choice is *penicillin* in a single dose of 4.8 million units. Alternate antibiotics are considered in the discussion of upper genital tract gonococcal infections (p. 144). In the child or senile woman, *estrogen* was formerly used to thicken the vaginal epithelium.

The pili of the cell wall of the gonococcus have been used to produce a vaccine, which is currently being tested as a serologic treatment for gonorrhea.

Bartholinitis is often of gonococcal origin but it commonly represents a secondary infection with *coliform* organisms or *polymicrobial* pathogens. In 15% of cases, *Bacteroides fragilis* may be recovered. Treatment of the acute infection includes antibiotics, analgesics, and heat. An *abscess* of the Bartholin gland presents as a painful, ovoid, tender mass in the inferior portion of the labia. Treatment is *incision* and *drainage*. An abscess may subside to form a *cyst,* which may be treated by *excision,* or more commonly, *marsupialization* (evacuation of the contents of the cyst and suturing its edges to those of the external incision).

Vaginitis is often *secondary* to vulvitis or cervicitis. *Atrophic vaginitis* occurs after natural or surgical menopause as a result of a deficiency of estrogens. It produces an irritating discharge, with pruritus, edema, and often dyspareunia. The pale, thin, smooth vaginal mucosa may be secondarily infected with *H. vaginalis* or *trichomonads*, which may cause a purulent or sanguineous discharge. Women who continue regular coitus are less likely to have atrophic vaginitis. Treatment is local application of *estrogen cream*.

The main causes of adult vaginitis are *Trichomonas, Candida*, and *nonspecific organisms*. Infections with *Trichomonas* and *Candida* occasionally occur together.

Trichomonas produces a thin, watery, yellowish-green, *foamy, malodorous* discharge. The organism is a flagellated protozoon, which may be identified in a *hanging-drop* preparation. It is transmitted, in part at least, through *sexual contact*. The hyperemic vaginal mucosa may exhibit *petechiae* (strawberry-like appearance) and cause pruritus and soreness. Manifestations of trichomoniasis are often aggravated after a menstrual period. The best treatment is *metronidazole* (Flagyl) 250 mg by mouth three times a day for seven days. A single dose of 2 g of metronidazole has also been found to be effective. It is occasionally necessary to treat the sexual partner as well.

Candida (*Monilia*) produces a thick, white, cheesy, *curdlike discharge*. On microscopic examination or culture the *yeastlike* buds and hyphae are seen. The infection may produce vulvar irritation, burning, and pruritus. *Exacerbation* of the infection is often noted in *pregnancy*, in *diabetes*, and with the use of *oral contraceptives* or *antibiotics*. The usual therapy is intravaginal insertion of *nystatin* (Mycostatin), *miconazole nitrate*, or *clotrimazole* in the form of cream or tablet, daily for seven days. *Gentian violet* (2%) is an older nonspecific treatment that is effective but less popular because it stains skin and underclothing.

Nonspecific vaginal discharge is diagnosed by the *exclusion* of other agents. *Hemophilus* organisms are often causative or contributory. *Ampicillin* and *tetracycline* are the drugs of choice; intravaginal *sulfa creams* are of value also. Antiseptic douches are of limited value. The vagina is normally *acidic* because of the lactic acid produced by action of lactobacilli (Döderlein bacillus) on glycogen.

In the investigation of a vaginal discharge, *foreign bodies* should be sought and removed. Although any severe vaginal infection may lead to a *bloody discharge, carcinoma must be excluded* by appropriate diagnostic techniques.

Pediatric vaginitis is commonly initiated by a foreign body. Additional predisposing factors are *poor hygiene* and *labial agglutination,* which is treated with *estrogen cream.* The organisms frequently involved are *Enterobius vermicularis* (pinworm), *Trichomonas vaginalis,* gonococci, and coliform bacilli. Pinworms may be identified with scotch tape and treated with *piperazine citrate.*

Microscopic demonstration of *chronic inflammatory cells* in the adult human cervix is virtually a *normal* finding. *Gonorrhea* produces an *acute cervicitis,* which may cause a profuse *purulent discharge* as well as a *chronic* infection; the frequently associated *urethritis* causes dysuria and frequency.

A *nonspecific cervicitis* may be related to *erosion* (ulceration of the everted columnar epithelium of the endocervix and the squamous epithelium of the portio vaginalis) or *eversion* (rolling out of the endocervical mucosa onto the portio). *Epidermidalization* (covering or replacement of columnar epithelium by stratified squamous epithelium) and plugging of endocervical glandular ducts may cause *retention cysts* (nabothian follicles). Chronic cervicitis is the *most common* cause of *leukorrhea*. Less common causes of cervicitis include secondary infection of a cervical chancre or a tuberculous or herpetic lesion.

Before treatment is begun for any cervicitis, a *Papanicolaou smear* should be obtained. Gonorrheal cervicitis is treated by systemic *penicillin* or an alternative antibiotic (p. 144). Nonspecific cervicitis may be treated by locally applied antibiotics, *cauterization,* or *cryosurgical removal* of infected tissue.

Endometritis usually points to an *underlying* cause. The principal associated lesions are submucous *myomas, endometrial polyps, carcinoma* of the endometrium, fragments of retained *placenta,* or a *foreign body.* The inflammatory reaction associated with an intrauterine device does not usually produce a clinical endometritis.

Pelvic inflammatory disease (P.I.D.), acute or chronic, is most commonly caused by the *gonococcus* (*Neisseria gonorrhoeae*). The other principal causes are *pyogenic, polymicrobial,* and *granulomatous* infections. Common organisms in the polymicrobial flora are aerobic and anaerobic streptococci, coliform bacilli, and anaerobes including *Bacteroides fragilis*. Gonorrheal P.I.D. is an *ascending* infection that spreads along *mucous membranes* from the vulva to the adnexa.

In the adult, gonococcal infection skips from *Skene's* glands, the *urethra*, and *Bartholin's glands* to the cervix, because the stratified squamous epithelium of the adult is rather resistant to the infection. In infants, however, a gonococcal vaginitis may be a rapidly progressive and highly contagious infection. Since the endometrium usually resists gonorrheal infection, the disease skips from the cervix to involve the *tube*, the main site of serious P.I.D. If untreated, the course of tubal infection is as follows: *acute, subacute*, and *chronic salpingitis*, which may progress to a *pyosalpinx* as the fimbriated end is blocked. Resorption of the pus converts the pyosalpinx to a *hydrosalpinx*. In advanced infection, the ovary, which may be adherent to the tube, is involved in a *perioophoritis*. In the final stages of the disease a *tubo-ovarian abscess* may form, in which a pus-filled cavity is surrounded by a common wall of tubal and ovarian tissue.

When the diagnosis of gonorrhea is made or suspected, a *serologic test for syphilis* should be performed at the same time and *repeated* several weeks later.

In patients with acute pelvic inflammatory disease, *temperature, leukocyte count*, and *sedimentation rate* are elevated. A marked rise in temperature requires a *blood culture*. *Radiologic examination* of the abdomen may be required to rule out ileus or mechanical intestinal obstruction. In pelvic inflammatory disease the pain and tenderness are usually located *lower* than in an acute abdomen of other cause and the *gastrointestinal* signs and symptoms are *less* prominent. Tachycardia, rigidity, and rebound are nonspecific, but an *adnexal mass* and *pain on motion of the cervix* suggest pelvic inflammatory disease, which often is exacerbated during the *menses*.

The *differential diagnosis* of salpingitis includes all forms of the acute abdomen. With *salpingitis* the pain is more likely *bilateral* and there is *less nausea and vomiting* than with appendicitis, for example. With ectopic pregnancy the leukocyte count, sedimentation rate, and temperature are lower and the patient may show signs of pregnancy (p. 80). When the peritonitis is caused by salpingitis the patient appears *less ill* than when the acute abdomen is a result of appendicitis or pancreatitis, for example.

In the diagnosis of the acute abdomen it is most important to distinguish pelvic inflammatory disease from the other causes, since acute *salpingitis* (like acute pyelonephritis) is a *nonsurgical* disease, which responds to *antibiotic* therapy, as opposed to ectopic pregnancy, appendicitis, and torsion of an adnexal mass, for example. Where *doubt* about a "surgical abdomen" persists, *laparotomy* must be performed. If the diagnosis proves wrong and acute salpingitis is found, the *abdomen* should be *closed* without further procedures.

Because of the *rapid spread* of pelvic inflammatory disease, it is appropriate to *treat gonorrhea* of the lower genitourinary tract *before confirmation* of the diagnosis is obtained. The standard treatment is 4.8 million units of *aqueous procaine penicillin G* in two intramuscular injections. One gram of *probenecid,* given at least 30 minutes before the antibiotic, prolongs the high blood level of penicillin. An alternative to aqueous penicillin is 3.5 g of *ampicillin* orally, preceded by 1 g of probenecid.

In cases of sensitivity to penicillin, *spectinomycin* (Trobicin) may be given in a dose of 2 g in a single intramuscular injection. Spectinomycin is recommended primarily for patients who are not cured with other antibiotics or who are likely to be infected with beta-lactamase-producing strains. A third possibility, except in the pregnant patient, is *tetracycline* (1.5 g by mouth followed by 0.5 g four times a day until a total of 9 g is given).

Gonococcal proctitis may require larger doses of antibiotics, either 2.4 million units of aqueous procaine penicillin G for five days by daily intramuscular injection, or 2 g of ampicillin trihydrate daily for five days. The treatment of choice may be spectinomycin hydrochloride, 4 g intramuscularly. Five days of penicillin therapy will cure incubating syphilis. If, however, the patient is treated with spectinomycin, which does not cure syphilis, the blood test for syphilis should be repeated.

The treatment of choice in *pelvic inflammatory disease* is penicillin, 10 to 15 million units per day intravenously, supplemented by other antibiotics that are effective against gram-negative infections. *Disseminated gonococcal infection* requires 6 to 12 million units of penicillin per day intravenously, followed by prolonged therapy with *ampicillin* or *amoxicillin*, 2 g daily for 10 to 14 days, after acute signs and symptoms have subsided. *Penicillin-allergic* patients are best treated with *tetracycline*.

Chronic pelvic inflammatory disease is often suspected on the basis of a history of *repetitive acute* infections. If the disease is untreated, the tubes are ultimately occluded and the mucosa and fimbriae are destroyed. The patient is thus rendered *infertile*. When antibiotic therapy is inadequate to eradicate the inflammation, a *follicular salpingitis* may result. This lesion predisposes to *ectopic pregnancy* (p. 80). In exacerbations of pelvic inflammatory disease and in the chronic form, polymicrobial infections with anaerobic organisms are often found.

The signs and symptoms of chronic pelvic inflammatory disease are referable primarily to the adnexal disease. Exacerbation of the infection leads to *adhesions, more or less constant pelvic pain,* and *dyspareunia*. A palpable *mass* and recurring *spikes of temperature* suggest a *tubo-ovarian abscess* or a *pelvic abscess*.

The important surgical decision in chronic pelvic inflammatory disease is *whether* or *when* to *operate* rather than *what* procedure to perform, for in most cases *total abdominal hysterectomy with bilateral salpingo-oophorectomy* is the operation of choice for the advanced lesion. The decision to operate therefore depends upon the *symptoms* and the degree of *incapacitation*. The possibility that an adnexal mass represents an *ovarian neoplasm* must be excluded by the appropriate diagnostic method. The differential diagnosis of chronic pelvic inflammatory disease also includes *ectopic pregnancy* and *endometriosis*.

The sudden disappearance of a mass accompanied by softening of the abdomen suggests rupture of a tubo-ovarian abscess. This emergency requires total hysterectomy and bilateral salpingo-oophorectomy. An abscess that points in the cul-de-sac may occasionally be drained by colpotomy, but a true tubo-ovarian abscess cannot be approached safely through that route. Pelvic inflammatory disease is occasionally accompanied by septic shock. The management is the same as that of septic shock of other causes (p. 79).

Particularly in the young patient, conservative surgical procedures are often attempted. Rarely, however, can a tube involved in gonococcal salpingitis be reconstructed sufficiently to ensure fertility, especially if the fimbriae are destroyed.

Active gonococcal infection in the mother may lead to gonococcal ophthalmia in the newborn. For prophylaxis, silver nitrate, penicillin, or occasionally another antibiotic is placed in the conjunctival sacs of all newborn infants as a routine.

Pyogenic infections caused by streptococci and staphylococci were formerly more common complications of abortion and delivery. Unlike gonorrhea, they spread by lymphatic and hematogenous routes. The infection extends directly through the endometrium and the myometrium into the parametria and broad ligaments, causing a pelvic cellulitis and involving the tube from the outside. In these infections also, the involved organs are occasionally secondarily invaded by coliform organisms. The pyogenic salpingitides usually respond to large doses of penicillin.

The granulomatous salpingitides are exemplified by tuberculosis, which still accounts for a small percentage of all pelvic inflammatory disease in the United States. The infection is almost always secondary to pulmonary tuberculosis. Tuberculous pelvic inflammatory disease is a hematogenous infection that involves the tube as the primary site in the pelvis. The abdominal end of the tube may remain open, although the fimbriae are often destroyed and peristalsis is abolished. Histologically the highly proliferative lesion may superficially resemble carcinoma. Peritoneal tuberculosis may be accompanied by ascites.

The infection involves primarily women between the ages of 20 and 40 and is characterized by malaise, a low-grade fever, and nagging abdominal pain. Menstrual disorders and infertility are common. Tuberculosis should be suspected in a case of salpingitis that does not respond to penicillin and in pelvic inflammatory disease in virgins. A granuloma on endometrial biopsy directs suspicion to the lesion, and the presence of acid-fast bacilli on a Ziehl-Neelsen stained preparation of the tissue is confirmatory. Final diagnosis is made by inoculation into guinea pigs.

When surgical extirpation was the mainstay of treatment, postoperative complications such as fistulas were common. Antituberculous drugs are now the treatment of choice. Chemotherapy is usually continued for 9 to 18 months, with surgical treatment reserved for an adnexal mass (to rule out carcinoma of the ovary) and for unresponsive pain or fever.

The primary drugs used for treatment of pelvic tuberculosis are streptomycin, ethambutol or para-aminosalicylic acid (PAS), and isoniazid (INH). Rifampicin (rifampin) is occasionally used instead of streptomycin.

An unusual form of chronic salpingitis is called salpingitis isthmica nodosa, which causes fibrosis of the tubal wall with nodular thickenings and obstruction at the cornual end. The cause of this lesion is poorly understood.

Pelvic Relaxation and Gynecologic Injuries

Pelvic relaxation refers to a group of anatomic, sometimes symptomatic, defects including *uterine prolapse* (*descensus*), relaxation of the anterior vaginal wall (*urethrocele* and *cystocele*), relaxation of the posterior wall (*rectocele*), herniation of the peritoneum of the cul-de-sac (*enterocele*), and *laceration* of the *perineum*. These disorders are usually related to childbirth or *aging* and are rarely congenital. Prolapse of the vagina may occur after hysterectomy.

The principal *weakness* is in the *endopelvic fascia* and the muscular *levator sling*. Attenuation of the *vesicovaginal* (anterior) portion of the endopelvic fascia, between bladder and anterior vaginal wall, results in *prolapse of the bladder* into the anterior vaginal wall (cystocele). Weakening of the connective tissue between the *urethra* and vagina produces a urethrocele. Weakening of the *rectovaginal* (posterior) portion of the endopelvic fascia causes bulging of the anterior wall of the *rectum* into the vagina (rectocele).

Laceration or attenuation of the condensed pericervical areolar tissue (endopelvic fascia), laceration of the perineum, and injury to the levator sling usually result from *obstetric injuries or the atrophy of aging.* Attenuation of the *cardinal* and *uterosacral ligaments* contributes to the relaxation. Herniation of *small bowel* through the hiatus between the uterosacral ligaments produces an *enterocele,* which is a *true hernia.* The components of pelvic relaxation occur in various degrees and combinations. The best *prevention* is good *obstetric care.*

The syndrome of pelvic relaxation is related in part to the anatomic changes associated with the bipedal condition. Women with pelvic relaxation are more likely than the general population to develop hemorrhoids, hernias, and varicose veins. Racial factors also play a role in susceptibility to pelvic relaxation. Black women, for example, are less likely than white women to develop uterine prolapse.

The greater prevalence of uterine prolapse in England as compared with the United States, however, is more likely related to differences in obstetric practice. Good obstetric management includes the appropriate use of elective (prophylactic) forceps and episiotomy, shortening of the second stage, and anatomic repair of lacerations. These maneuvers protect the perivaginal connective tissues and the muscles of the pelvic floor.

The relative roles of the pelvic musculature and the connective tissue ligaments in the prevention of pelvic relaxation remain somewhat controversial. The levator ani, which consists of the pubococcygeus, iliococcygeus, and ischiococcygeus, forms the deep support. The perineal muscles form a second line of defense; they comprise the ischiocavernosus, bulbocavernosus, and superficial and deep transverse perineal muscles, together with the urogenital diaphragm and external anal sphincter. The broad ligament provides no support, but the condensed connective tissue in the cardinal and uterosacral ligaments helps to maintain the uterus in its normal position.

The signs and symptoms of pelvic relaxation depend on the combination and degree of anatomic defects. *Uterine prolapse* usually produces merely a *sagging sensation* in the pelvis.

Severe degrees of prolapse are associated with other symptomatic components of pelvic relaxation.

In first-degree prolapse, the uterus descends but the cervix remains within the vagina. In second-degree prolapse, the cervix appears partially or totally outside the vaginal orifice. In third-degree prolapse (procidentia), the entire uterus is outside the vaginal orifice. In a prolapsed uterus the cervix is often hypertrophied and ulcerated, but is not more frequently subject to carcinoma.

A *cystocele* may reach large size without becoming symptomatic. Problems referable to a cystocele include *frequency of urination*, a sensation of *pelvic pressure*, and a predisposition to recurrent *urinary tract infections*. The cystocele does *not*, however, produce *stress incontinence* (the involuntary loss of urine upon increase in intraabdominal pressure).

A *rectocele* causes a *sensation of a mass* in the vagina and *difficulty in evacuating the rectum* except by placing a hand in the vagina to reduce the bulge. The *enterocele* is subject to all the *complications of hernias* elsewhere in the body. The *relaxed perineum* may lead to unsatisfactory intercourse.

The most serious complaint in patients with pelvic relaxation is *stress incontinence*, which results from a *urethrocele*, or a *funneling of the bladder neck*.

Differential diagnosis of pelvic relaxation usually presents few problems. A prolapsed uterus must be differentiated from a normally situated uterus with an elongated cervix. An enterocele must be differentiated from a high rectocele, a urethrocele from a suburethral diverticulum, and a cystocele from a large midline mesonephric ductal cyst.

The *treatment* of pelvic relaxation depends on *correction* of the *fascial and muscular defects*. The *cystocele* is repaired by plication of the anterior portion of the endopelvic fascia (*anterior colporrhaphy*, p. 134). Care must be taken to *avoid overcorrection*, thereby obliterating the posterior urethrovesical angle and producing *stress incontinence*. An extensive anterior colporrhaphy should be accompanied by a *plication of the bladder neck* (Kelly plication, p. 134) to maintain the *urethrovesical angle.*

The *rectocele* is repaired by plication of the posterior portion of the endopelvic fascia (*posterior colporrhaphy,* p. 134). In complete pelvic repairs, it is desirable to perform only *minimal posterior colporrhaphy* in a young woman in order to *preserve sexual function.* A relaxed perineum may be reconstructed to provide normal support by the operation known as *perineorrhaphy.* An *enterocele* is repaired by *excision of the hernial sac* and *obliteration of the hiatus* between the uterosacral ligaments.

Retroversion, except possibly the adherent variety found in endometriosis (p. 156), is a *normal variant* of uterine position. It does not require surgical therapy.

The *abdominal approach* to correction of pelvic relaxation is anatomically *illogical* and therapeutically *unsuccessful.* The principal treatment of *uterine prolapse* is *vaginal hysterectomy.* This procedure in itself, however, does not correct the often accompanying cystocele and rectocele or the stress incontinence. These problems are managed by *colporrhaphy* and *Kelly plication* (p. 134). The advantages of vaginal hysterectomy are the *prevention of pregnancy,* which could break down a previously successful repair, and *removal* of a *functionless organ,* which could be the site of benign or malignant disease.

Before vaginal hysterectomy and repair of a cystocele it is desirable to eradicate local infections of the vagina, cervix, and bladder. For minor degrees of pelvic relaxation, exercises to strengthen the perineal muscles may be helpful.

Pessaries are rarely used today, except for temporary replacement of a prolapsed uterus during preoperative healing of an infected cervix. They may be used also as a therapeutic test to ascertain whether repositioning of the uterus will relieve the patient's symptoms. Pessaries are used for definitive treatment only in the aged patient or the woman who is too sick to tolerate a surgical procedure. Pessaries may be associated with an increased incidence of vaginal carcinoma.

The Manchester operation (p. 134) is an unpopular alternative to vaginal hysterectomy in this country. In a Manchester procedure the cardinal ligaments are plicated but the uterus is not removed. It is justified only in the patient with symptomatic prolapse who desires further childbearing. The operation may be complicated by the development of an incompetent cervix (p. 78) and the need for subsequent delivery by cesarean section.

Stress incontinence of urine is the most troublesome result of pelvic relaxation. It may become sufficiently serious to render the patient a *social invalid.* It is caused primarily by *blunting* of the *posterior urethrovesical* angle, which is normally 90 to 100 degrees. The basic defect is *weakness* of the *musculofascial supports* of the *bladder neck* and upper urethra. Urinary continence depends on maintenance of a *posterior urethrovesical angle,* normal *detrusor function,* and support by the *muscles of the pelvic floor*.

Urination begins with contraction of the detrusor and funneling of the bladder neck. With voluntary increase in intravesical pressure the pelvic floor relaxes and urination occurs. With stress incontinence the posterior urethrovesical angle is blunted and the patient is always in the first stage of urination.

Type I stress incontinence results when the posterior urethrovesical angle is obliterated but the urethral axis retains its normal relation to the vagina. Further descent of the anterior wall of the vagina causes descent of the base of the bladder and rotation of the urethral axis backward and downward. When these anatomic changes are superimposed on loss of the posterior urethrovesical angle, Type II stress incontinence results.

The *differential diagnosis* of urinary incontinence includes *stress, urgency, overflow,* and *true incontinence.* With *stress* incontinence usually a *small amount* of urine is produced when intraabdominal pressure is increased, as with coughing or sneezing. Tumors may cause temporary stress incontinence, which disappears when the lesions are removed. *True incontinence* most often results from a urinary tract *fistula* (p. 133), which causes more or less *constant loss* of urine.

Urgency results from *hypertonia* of the *detrusor*. In this condition *large amounts* of urine are voided. Urgency may be produced by urinary tract *infection* and vaginitis (infectious or atrophic). Eradication of the infection and local estrogen may be beneficial. *Overflow* incontinence results from *overdistension* of the bladder. Underlying causes include *neuropathies*, as with diabetes mellitus, syphilis, multiple sclerosis, and spinal injuries. Accurate diagnosis of urinary incontinence requires a careful history of symptoms, pelvic and neurologic examinations, and urinary cultures and sensitivities.

Additional diagnostic studies include measurement of residual urine to rule out inadequate emptying and a neuropathy involving the bladder. Urethrocystoscopy and cystometrograms provide objective evidence of intrinsic lesions of the urinary tract and of the relations of bladder neck and urethra to the vagina. These techniques thus aid in the identification of Type I and Type II stress incontinence. Intravenous pyelography may be required to rule out an ectopic ureter and other lesions higher in the urinary tract.

The Kelly plication (p. 134) is the mainstay of surgical treatment of Type I stress incontinence. For cure of Type II, a retropubic suspension of the bladder neck (Marshall-Marchetti procedure, p. 134), with or without Kelly plication, may be required.

When the Kelly plication (vaginal approach) and the retropubic suspension of the bladder neck (abdominal approach) are unsuccessful, one of the many "sling" operations may be effective. In these procedures a sling of rectus fascia or synthetic material is passed under the urethra through the space of Retzius and reattached to the anterior abdominal wall. Reduction in weight and treatment of a chronic cough will improve the results of surgical management of stress incontinence.

Total incontinence of urine may be caused by fistulas between the vagina and the urinary tract. These lesions are the result of the close anatomic relation of the female reproductive and urinary organs. The obstetric causes have decreased relatively as a result of technical improvements and the avoidance of difficult vaginal deliveries and long labors, but the gynecologic injuries have increased relatively as a result of more extensive surgical and radiologic treatment.

Vesicovaginal fistulas may result from unrecognized injury during hysterectomy or colporrhaphy. If not repaired immediately, these fistulas are most successfully closed, usually by the vaginal route, after a delay of four to six months. Other causes are injury from radiation and direct involvement by carcinoma.

A vesicovaginal fistula may be demonstrated by the appearance of dye in the vagina after instillation of methylene blue into the bladder. A ureterovaginal fistula may result from a radical (p. 133) or difficult total hysterectomy in which the ureter is ligated or cut. This fistula may be demonstrated by the appearance of dye in the vagina after intravenous injection of indigo carmine or by pyelography. A urethrovaginal fistula distal to the bladder neck is unlikely to result in urinary incontinence and ordinarily requires no treatment.

Vaginal fistulas may involve the bowel as well as the urinary tract. A rectovaginal fistula may result from unrecognized obstetric injuries, gynecologic operations, radiation therapy, or direct growth of a carcinoma. A small rectovaginal fistula may result only in incontinence of gas, whereas a larger fistula usually causes fecal incontinence as well. The principles of closure are similar to those of vesicovaginal fistulas.

Adenomyosis and Endometriosis

Adenomyosis and *endometriosis* are frequently discussed together although they are etiologically different disorders, which require different treatments.

Adenomyosis is a condition in which endometrial tissue penetrates the myometrium by *direct extension* from the lining of the uterine cavity. The circumscribed lesion is termed an *adenomyoma* and the diffuse form *adenomyosis*.

Endometriosis is a disorder in which endometrial tissue occurs outside its normal intrauterine location *not connected* with the endometrial surface. It also may be a circumscribed (*endometrioma*) or diffuse (*endometriosis*) lesion.

Diagnosis of adenomyosis requires the finding of endometrial glands or stroma a specified distance from the base of the endometrium. This distance varies, according to different authorities, from one high-power to two low-power fields. One low-power field, however, is a commonly accepted definition.

Adenomyosis comprises endometrial tissue surrounded by myometrium. In special circumstances, gland or stroma may predominate or occur exclusively. Since the tissue is composed largely of basal endometrium, it is not fully responsive to the endocrine changes of the endometrial cycle or to exogenously administered hormones.

Adenomyosis, unlike endometriosis, is most common in *multiparas* in the *fourth to sixth decades*. It may be associated with *myomas* and *endometrial hyperplasia* and occasionally with *endometriosis* and *carcinoma of the endometrium*. Grossly, the myometrium is irregularly *thickened* on cut surface.

The characteristic symptoms and signs of adenomyosis are *progressive dysmenorrhea, menorrhagia,* and an *enlarging tender uterus.* Additional findings include dyspareunia and a premenstrual syndrome that resembles pelvic congestion (p. 258). The *diagnosis* is often made *incidentally* at the time of laparotomy. The differential diagnosis includes carcinoma of the corpus, endometrial polyps, and myomas. The gross pathologic differential diagnosis includes *sarcoma* and *myoma*. Unlike the myoma, neither the adenomyoma nor the sarcoma has a pseudocapsule that allows easy enucleation from the surrounding myometrium.

A special form of the lesion is stromal adenomyosis, or endometrial stromatosis. This disease may clinically resemble a low-grade endometrial sarcoma.

The etiologic factors in adenomyosis are unknown, although an *estrogenic imbalance* may be influential.

The incidence of the disease is difficult to assess, although it is commonly found in uteri removed for other causes. Since *hormonal treatment* is generally *unsatisfactory,* the symptomatic lesion is most often treated by *hysterectomy*. In women near the *menopause,* after malignant disease has been excluded, *temporization* may be logical, for the lesion regresses with cessation of ovarian function.

The prevalence of *endometriosis* is difficult to ascertain because it also is often discovered as an *incidental* finding at laparotomy. It is most commonly found in *nulliparas* between the ages of *30 and 40*. The widespread use of *laparoscopy* has resulted in the detection of many more examples of endometriosis recently. It is said to occur more commonly in the white, middle-class, high-income patients who marry late. These differences most likely reflect *socioeconomic* rather than racial factors. Private patients, furthermore, are more likely to register minor complaints, thereby creating the impression of a greater prevalence of the disease in that group.

Endometriosis is *not* found in the *prepuberal* girl or in the *postmenopausal* period and seems to be improved during pregnancy. *Early childbearing* plays a role in *preventing* endometriosis.

Several etiologic concepts are still being debated. One hypothesis favors retgrograde menstruation, with the resulting implantation of endometrial tissue on the ovaries and peritoneum. A retroverted uterus, which is commonly found in patients with endometriosis, may predispose to retrograde menses. A second etiologic hypothesis is celomic metaplasia, by which celomic derivatives are transformed into tissues of endometrial type. A third concept, which combines retrograde menses with metaplasia, is induction, by means of which a chemical substance from sloughed endometrial tissue leads to transformation of other tissues to the endometrial type. Hematogenous and lymphatic spread probably plays only a small role in the histogenesis of endometriosis.

Endometriosis usually comprises both *gland* and *stroma*, although one or the other element may be predominant or exclusively present. The gross lesions may resemble "powder burns" on the peritoneum and serosal surfaces. Large hemorrhagic cysts of the ovary containing dark blood are referred to as *"chocolate cysts,"* although not all such hemorrhagic ovarian cysts are the result of endometriosis.

When the wall of a hemorrhagic cyst contains hemosiderin but the epithelium of origin is unidentifiable, the diagnosis should be hemorrhagic cyst rather than endometrial cyst.

Rupture of an endometrial cyst may lead to extensive *adhesions,* denser than those of pelvic inflammatory disease. Intraperitoneal bleeding or pain resulting from rupture of an endometrioma may create a surgical emergency. The resulting adhesions may cause *fixed retroversion* of the uterus, involvement of adjacent organs, and *strictures* of the *bowel.* In extreme cases, a "frozen pelvis" may result.

The structures involved in endometriosis, in order of frequency, are the *ovary, the posterior cul-de-sac, the uterosacral ligaments, the rectovaginal septum,* the oviducts, the rectosigmoid, and the bladder. Distant organs are rarely involved. Endometriosis of the lymph nodes, umbilicus, pleura, and extremities is difficult to explain on the basis of the common histogenetic theories.

Carcinoma may develop in ovarian endometriosis, but unless a clear transition from normal endometrium to malignant tissue is seen within the ovary, the origin of the tumor from endometriosis cannot be proved.

The endometriotic tissue is usually *responsive* to the *hormones* of the menstrual cycle and to externally supplied hormones. This endocrine dependence explains the progress of the disease as well as the response to treatment.

The *accuracy* of *preoperative diagnosis* of endometriosis is relatively *low.* The lesion is often found incidentally in patients operated upon for other reasons. The number of false-positive and false-negative diagnoses will be reduced by preoperative *culdoscopy* or *laparoscopy. Definitive diagnosis* is made only after *histologic examination* of a *biopsy* specimen.

Endometriosis characteristically presents with *acquired dysmenorrhea,* acute and chronic *pelvic pain,* and abnormal *uterine bleeding. Infertility* may become a major problem. The dysmenorrhea, beginning in the third or fourth decade, is *progressive.* As the disease continues, pain and bleeding occur in increasingly greater portions of the menstrual cycle. *Dyspareu-*

nia may result from involvement of the uterosacral ligaments and implants in the cul-de-sac and fornices. The abnormal bleeding may result from *ovarian dysfunction*, which together with *dense adhesions* may lead to infertility.

Less common manifestations of endometriosis include pain, bleeding with bowel movements or tenesmus (as a result of involvement of the rectovaginal septum and rectum), and dysuria and cyclic hematuria (as a result of involvement of the bladder). A less specific but more common manifestation is dull pain radiating to the thighs.

An accurate *rectovaginal examination* is essential for the diagnosis of endometriosis. Highly suggestive findings include *nodules* in the *cul-de-sac*, the *posterior fornix*, and the *uterosacral ligament; fixed retroversion* of the uterus; and *obliteration* of the *cul-de-sac* by *dense adhesions*. *Differential diagnosis* includes chronic *pelvic inflammatory disease* and *ovarian neoplasms*. Additional diseases to be considered are *carcinoma of the rectum or sigmoid, diverticulitis*, and *tuberculosis*. With endometriosis a greater degree of *fixation* of organs is found than with other diseases that are considered in differential diagnosis. Laboratory data are not diagnostic, but a normal white count and sedimentation rate point to endometriosis rather than pelvic inflammatory disease.

Pelvic examination under anesthesia may differentiate endometriosis from the pelvic congestion syndrome, since in endometriosis the thickening and nodularity of the uterosacral ligaments, for example, will not decrease or disappear. The diagnostic workup, depending on signs and symptoms, may include barium enema, cystoscopy, and intravenous pyelography.

Treatment of endometriosis is influenced by the patient's age and parity. The three methods of management are *palliative, hormonal*, and *surgical*. Palliation (conservative therapy) entails careful observation, reassurance, and analgesics. A trial of *pregnancy*, where possible, should be recommended, for it may be curative. Observation is *contraindicated* in the presence of an *undiagnosed adnexal mass*.

Surgical and hormonal techniques of management of endometriosis are *complementary*. Prolonged hormonal therapy, which is time-consuming and expensive, should be reserved for patients in whom there is a *histologic diagnosis* of endometriosis.

Surgical therapy is indicated for *failure* of *medical management, persistent infertility* for one year after hormonal treatment, and *ovarian masses* greater than 6 cm in diameter. Surgical therapy may also be the modality of choice when the patient has *completed her family* or is *near the menopause*. Surgical management may range from conservative procedures, such as excision of small implants, to total abdominal hysterectomy and bilateral salpingo-oophorectomy with removal of as many of the implants as possible.

Total abdominal hysterectomy and bilateral salpingo-oophorectomy are often curative even when not all of the implants are removed. It is unwise to attempt excision of every implant when adjacent organs would thereby be jeopardized. Hysterectomy without removal of the adnexa may be performed in a young patient who has completed her family. After hysterectomy and removal of the adnexa it is possible to provide hormonal supplementation, since there is no longer a proliferating endometrial mucosa to generate additional endometriotic implants.

In connection with conservative operations, uterine suspension and presacral neurectomy may be performed for symptomatic relief. Further decrease in pain may be achieved by interruption of the nerve tracts in the uterosacral ligaments.

The *hormonal* control of endometriosis is often the treatment of choice. Hormonal therapy is indicated in patients who *refuse operations;* it is, furthermore, *adjunctive* to conservative *operations. Estrogens, androgens,* and *progestins* have all been used to interrupt the ovarian cycle and control endometriosis.

Almost any estrogen may be employed successfully, although it may be unwise to administer diethylstilbestrol to patients in the childbearing age when the steroidal estrogens provide an acceptable alternative. Androgens are also effective but they carry the theoretic danger of masculinization. Methyl testosterone in doses of 5 mg every day for three to six months, however, rarely produces permanent side effects.

The mainstays of current hormonal therapy of endometriosis are the synthetic steroids used commonly as oral contraceptives. The *progestins* in these preparations produce a *pseudopregnancy,* characterized by atrophy of the endometrial glands and decidual transformation of the stroma.

Almost any of the currently used oral contraceptives may be employed for treatment of endometriosis, but excellent results have been achieved over long periods of time with norethynodrel and mestranol (Enovid). The initial dose of 10 mg/day is gradually increased at two-week intervals to a maximum of 20 to 40 mg/day. Such therapy continued for nine months has resulted in cures or remissions in 80% of cases of endometriosis.

Hormonal therapy is commonly complicated by *nausea, edema, irregular uterine bleeding,* and possible *growth of myomas.* The hormones may also be used preoperatively to "soften" the adhesions in a patient about to undergo surgical treatment.

Progestins alone, either by mouth or intramuscular injection, have also been used successfully. Medroxyprogesterone acetate (Depo-Provera) is currently approved by the F.D.A. for use in endometriosis but not routine contraception. The injection may be given every two weeks in doses of 50 or 100 mg. If breakthrough bleeding occurs, the progestin is supplemented with estrogen by injection or by mouth.

Danazol, a derivative of ethisterone, is an orally effective agent that inhibits the anterior pituitary. It is anabolic and weakly androgenic. Its main side-effect is weight gain. The drug is required in doses of up to 800 mg/day for six months. The considerable expense of this new form of therapy is its major drawback. Unlike the progestational agents, which stimulate parts of the endometrium and produce a pseudopregnancy, danazol does not stimulate the target organ but produces a pseudomenopause.

Radiotherapy plays virtually no role in the modern management of endometriosis. It was formerly used to effect castration but the dense adhesions may jeopardize the adherent viscera, which are immobile in the field of radiation.

Gynecologic Tumors

Although neoplasms of the *breast* are treated by general surgeons in most parts of this country, the obstetrician-gynecologist has excellent opportunities to detect these lesions during *prenatal* visits, at the time of the annual *Papanicolaou smear,* and during examinations for *contraception.* The details of history of mammary disease and physical examination of the breast are given on pages 11–14. Because mammary carcinoma is the *most common cancer* in women, every mass in the breast must be viewed with suspicion. *Fixation, retraction,* and *asymmetry* of the breasts, as well as *discharge from the nipple,* require further diagnostic investigation. *Biopsy* should be performed by a surgeon competent and prepared to perform mastectomy under the same anesthetic.

Current recommendations regarding mammography are as follows:

1. Mammographic screening should be available to women over 50.
2. For women between the ages of 40 and 49, mammography should be used only for those who have had mammary cancer or whose mothers or sisters have had the disease.
3. For women between the ages of 35 and 39, mammography should be used only if the woman has previously had cancer in one breast.
4. The examination of the breast by heat (thermography) has proved to be less valuable than that by x-ray.
5. Mammography should not be used to screen women under the age of 35.
6. Mammography should be used for women of any age to aid in the diagnosis of suspected tumor.

The gynecologist is likely to encounter *three benign diseases* of the breast. An *intraductal papilloma* is the tumor that most commonly causes bleeding from the nipple. A *fibroadenoma* presents as a firm, discrete mass that requires biopsy to distinguish it from carcinoma. *Fibrocystic disease* poses diagnostic difficulties. The lesion presents as diffuse nodularity associated with increasing tenderness immediately before the menses. A nodule that does not regress postmenstrually may require biopsy. Fibrocystic disease is occasionally aggravated by *oral contraceptives*, particularly those with a high content of estrogen.

Benign tumors of the vulva include those of the skin in general and a few special growths. *Condyloma acuminatum* is *viral* rather than primarily neoplastic and is discussed among infections (p. 139). *Abscesses* and *cysts* of *Bartholin's gland* are discussed under inflammatory lesions (p. 140). Solid benign epithelial tumors include papillomas, adenomas, and nevi. Sebaceous cysts and hidradenomas are also found on the vulva.

The hidradenoma may be highly cellular and therefore mistaken for an adenocarcinoma but it is rarely malignant. Benign connective tissue tumors of the vulva include lipomas, fibromas, hemangiomas, and lymphangiomas. Varices of the vulva may be mistaken for neoplasms.

Any *suspicious* lesion of the vulva, particularly in older women, should be subjected to *biopsy*.

The International Society for the Study of Vulvar Disease has suggested a logical and succinct classification of the vulvar dystrophies (Table 7). Included among the vulvar dystrophies are disorders formerly described as leukoplakia, kraurosis,

TABLE 7. The Vulvar Dystrophies

I. Hyperplastic Dystrophy
   A. *Without atypia*
   B. *With atypia*
II. Lichen Sclerosus
III. Mixed Dystrophy (lichen sclerosus with foci of epithelial hyperplasia)
   A. *Without atypia*
   B. *With atypia*

atrophic dystrophy, hyperplastic vulvitis, leukoplakic vulvitis, and neurodermatitis. Additionally, the following terms are no longer recommended: lichen sclerosus et atrophicus, leukokeratosis, Bowen's disease, erythroplasia of Queyrat, and carcinoma simplex.

Dystrophic lesions are important because they are sometimes precursors of carcinoma of the vulva. *"White lesions"* of the vulva include a variety of disorders, only some of which are premalignant. The greater the *cellular atypia,* the more likely is a white lesion to be a precursor of carcinoma.

In hyperplastic dystrophy there is epithelial hyperplasia, acanthosis, hyperkeratosis, and chronic inflammation. In lichen sclerosus there is thinning of the squamous epithelium with loss of the rete pegs. The dermis just beneath the squamous epithelium looks acellular and homogeneous. In mixed dystrophy, areas of lichen sclerosus and hyperplastic dystrophy are found in the same lesion. The atypia accompanying any of the dystrophies may be classified as mild, moderate, or severe. Hyperkeratosis and parakeratosis may be found in all grades of atypia.

Atrophic lesions of the vulva may cause pruritus, which leads to scratching and secondary infection. Dystrophic lesions with cellular atypia may be precursors of vulvar carcinoma. Suspicious lesions should be subjected to biopsy. Widespread dysplastic lesions may be managed best by prophylactic vulvectomy.

Carcinoma of the vulva accounts for about 5% of all gynecologic cancers. The invasive lesion may be preceded by *dysplasia* and *carcinoma in situ.*

The typical vulvar carcinoma in situ is of the squamous cell variety. Another intraepithelial form, Paget's disease, which may be of apocrine origin, usually involves postmenopausal women. Pathognomonic Paget cells with clear, vacuolated cytoplasm are found, initially in the basal layers of the epidermis and later throughout the epithelium. Papanicolaou smears are unreliable for diagnosis of vulvar carcinoma because of the frequently associated hyperkeratosis. Toluidine blue may aid in selecting a site for the biopsy. Because these lesions are often multifocal, multiple biopsies are required to rule out invasion. The preinvasive lesion may be treated safely by simple vulvectomy. Paget's disease may recur in the vulva after local excision and may involve anus, cervix, and breasts.

Invasive carcinoma of the *vulva* is of the *squamous cell* variety in 95% of cases. It most frequently occurs in *postmenopausal* women but is occasionally found in younger women as well. About 40% of vulvar carcinomas are preceded by identifiable dysplastic lesions and intraepithelial carcinoma. Etiologic factors include *chronic infections* (such as lymphogranuloma venereum) and poor hygiene.

The most common sites of carcinoma of the vulva in order of frequency are the labium majus, the posterior commissure, the clitoris, and the labium minus. Spread occurs locally and lymphatic drainage is first to inguinal and femoral nodes and later to deep pelvic nodes.

Carcinoma of the vulva may present as a persistent asymptomatic exophytic *mass or ulcer* or may cause *pruritus,* a foul-smelling bloody *discharge,* or *pain* on urination or defecation. Diagnosis is provided by *biopsy,* which is the only means of distinguishing an intraepithelial from an early invasive lesion. Use of toluidine blue and colposcopy may aid in directing biopsy to the most abnormal areas. Because treatment of the two lesions varies greatly, *multiple biopsies* should be performed to rule out invasion. Differential diagnosis includes *syphilis* and other *granulomatous venereal* lesions.

Stage 0 is carcinoma in situ. Invasive carcinoma of the vulva, like other pelvic cancers, may be staged. Stage I lesions are confined to the vulva and are less than 2 cm in diameter. Inguinal nodes may or may not be palpable but are not enlarged or fixed. Stage II lesions are also confined to the vulva but are greater than 2 cm in diameter. Nodes may or may not be palpable but are not enlarged or fixed. Stage III lesions include tumors of any size with adjacent spread to the urethra, vagina, perineum, or anus; or palpable nodes in the groin that are enlarged, firm, and mobile (clinically suspect for metastases).

Stage IV lesions include tumors of any size that infiltrate the mucosa of the bladder or rectum, are fixed to bone, or have distant metastases.

Treatment of carcinoma of the vulva is *radical vulvectomy* (p. 134) with en bloc removal of *inguinal* and *femoral lymph nodes*. If the *superficial* nodes are *positive*, the *deep pelvic* nodes are dissected.

Conventional radiation is not effective treatment, but megavoltage therapy is occasionally employed for inoperable lesions or recurrences. The five-year survival rate in Stages I and II is about 75%. In Stage III it is 40%, and in Stage IV it is close to zero.

Basal cell carcinoma may be treated by wide local excision or simple vulvectomy without node dissection.

An adenocarcinoma of the vulva may arise rarely from Bartholin's gland. Secondary carcinomas of the vulva may represent metastases from a primary cancer of the uterus or rectum. Uncommon malignant tumors of the vulva include melanoma (pigmented and unpigmented), lymphoma, and fibrosarcoma.

Symptomatic *benign* lesions of the *vagina* are uncommon. *Inclusion cysts* are commonly 1 to 2 cm in diameter. They usually result from burial of tags of squamous epithelium under a suture line after episiotomy or repair of a laceration. Myomas and fibromas are rare lesions that produce no characteristic clinical findings. *Cysts of Gartner's duct* (mesonephric duct) may form in the upper portion of the vagina. *Endometriosis* of the vagina may produce dysmenorrhea and dyspareunia (p. 156).

Adenosis of the vagina develops from müllerian remnants. Administration of *diethylstilbestrol* (DES) to the mother during pregnancy has been associated with adenosis and *adenocarcinoma* of the vagina in the offspring. For this reason, DES is contraindicated in pregnancy. Children of mothers who have received the drug during pregnancy should be examined carefully to detect vaginal lesions.

The most important *carcinoma* of the vagina is of the *squa*-

mous cell variety, although it accounts for only 2% of female genital cancers. Spread occurs *locally* and by *lymphatics*. An intraepithelial form resembling that of the cervix often precedes invasive cancer. A *positive Papanicolaou* smear after hysterectomy suggests carcinoma of the vagina. Diagnosis is made by biopsy, often aided by Schiller's test and colposcopy.

The most common site for vaginal carcinoma is the posterior wall of the upper third of the vagina. The lesion may be exophytic or ulcerative. In advanced stages the vaginal tube may be fixed to the pelvic side wall. Carcinomas of the upper vagina may behave like those of the cervix, whereas those of the lowermost vagina spread like those of the vulva. Death is commonly from uremia.

Staging of carcinoma of the vagina resembles that of the cervix. Stage 0 is carcinoma in situ. Stage I carcinoma is limited to the vaginal wall. Stage II carcinoma extends into the paravaginal connective tissue but does not reach the pelvic side wall. A Stage III lesion reaches the pelvic side wall. Stage IV carcinoma involves the mucosa of the bladder or rectum (IVa) or has spread to distant organs (IVb). If squamous cell carcinoma is found in both cervix and vagina, it should be considered primary cancer of the cervix with extension.

Treatment of carcinoma of the vagina has not been satisfactorily standardized. Neither radiation nor surgical therapy has been highly successful. The five-year survival is still only 33%. Ultraradical operations may improve the cure rate slightly.

Carcinoma in the vagina is more often secondary than primary. The vagina is involved by direct spread from the cervix or by metastases from the ovaries, oviducts, choriocarcinoma, and occasionally carcinoma of the breast or hypernephroma. The vagina is involved by metastases, direct extension, or recurrence in about 10% of carcinomas of the corpus.

Sarcoma botryoides is a rare, highly malignant, usually fatal tumor that involves the vagina and is ordinarily found in infants.

Benign lesions of the cervix include polyps and condylomata acuminata (p. 139). *Polyps,* which may be single or multiple, have a core of connective tissue and an epithelial covering. They are usually *glandular,* arising from the endocervix, but are occasionally *squamous,* arising from the portio. They range in size from minute to several centimeters in length. They may cause *no symptoms* or may produce irregular *bleeding* or increased vaginal *discharge.* They very *rarely* undergo *malignant* change. A large polyp may be confused with a prolapsed myoma. The treatment is polypectomy, followed by fractional *curettage.*

Occasionally hyperplasia of the endocervical epithelium may result from the use of oral contraceptives. This change should not be confused with adenocarcinoma. This form of hyperplasia may produce contact bleeding but will regress after discontinuation of oral contraception.

Benign tumors of the cervix include leiomyomas, hemangiomas, and squamous papillomas. In addition, endometriosis and adenomyosis, as well as cysts and adenomas arising from mesonephric remnants, may involve the cervix. Adenosis and adenocarcinoma of the cervix, as well as of the vagina, have been reported in the children of mothers who received stilbestrol during their pregnancies.

Invasive carcinoma of the cervix is the *most common* cancer of the female genital tract, accounting for 50 to 65% of all gynecologic cancers. It is usually preceded by an *intraepithelial form,* which in turn is preceded by various degrees of increasing *dysplasia. Cervical intraepithelial neoplasia* (CIN) is a term that includes epithelial changes ranging from mild dysplasia to carcinoma in situ (CIS). All forms of cervical intraepithelial neoplasia may *regress,* but the earlier stages do so more commonly. The etiologic factors in dysplasia, carcinoma in situ, and invasive carcinoma are similar. The disease is apparently related to *poor genital hygiene* and *trauma* to the cervix. It is therefore more common in *lower socioeconomic* classes and women who begin *coitus* and *childbearing early* in their lives. It is also more common in prostitutes and other women with multiple sexual partners, particularly those with *poor penile hygiene.* Additional factors of etiologic importance include contact with Herpesvirus hominis type II (p. 140) and smegma, and, indirectly, lack of circumcision in the partners. Recent studies suggest that spermatozoa may be of primary etiologic significance. Carcinoma of the cervix is uncommon in Jewish women.

Dysplasia connotes nuclear atypia of the cervical epithelium without involvement of its entire thickness. True carcinoma in situ (intraepithelial, or preinvasive, cancer) usually involves the entire thickness of the cervical epithelium. The histologic changes include loss of polarity, hyperchromatism, abnormal mitoses, and increase in nuclear size and number of nucleoli.

The essential feature of intraepithelial carcinoma is the limitation of the abnormal cells by the basement membrane of the cervical epithelium. Involvement of the endocervical glands does not constitute invasion, because the glands are part of the cervical epithelium.

Microinvasion represents the transition between intraepithelial carcinoma and the invasive lesion. The definition and the treatment of this stage of the disease are still somewhat controversial, although the earliest forms are now often managed in the same manner as carcinoma in situ.

Histologically *most* carcinomas of the cervix (about 95%) are *squamous cell lesions*. About 5% are *adenocarcinomas;* carcinomas of mesonephric origin are rare. The tumor most commonly arises at the *squamocolumnar junction.* Chromosomal *aneuploidy* is found with increasing frequency as the lesion progresses from dysplasia through intraepithelial carcinoma to frankly invasive cancer. The tumor spreads *locally* into the *vagina* and *parametria* and then by regional *lymphatics*. A cervix that harbors an invasive lesion may be grossly normal, ulcerated, or replaced by a bulky exophytic tumor.

The peak incidence of *carcinoma in situ* occurs at about *37 years,* whereas that of *invasive* cancer occurs about ten years later (*45 to 48 years*). Because *clinical signs* of cervical cancer occur relatively *late,* success in the early detection and cure of this tumor depends on its identification in the *preclinical stages*. The most important means of achieving this goal is the routine use of the *Papanicolaou smear* (exfoliative cytology).

The earliest clinical signs of carcinoma of the cervix are *blood-tinged leukorrhea* and *postcoital* or *contact bleeding*. Pelvic pain, edema of the lower extremity (lymphatic involvement), irritability of the bladder, and rectal discomfort are *late* signs. Cachexia and genital tract fistulas indicate advanced disease. The tumor ultimately obstructs the ureters, producing *uremia*, the most common cause of *death* from carcinoma of the cervix. In advanced cases *infection* is often superimposed.

Successful management of carcinoma of the cervix depends on the detection of the *preinvasive lesion*, for intraepithelial carcinoma is curable in virtually 100% of cases. Once frank invasion occurs, the five-year cure rate drops to about 85%. The mainstay of detection of the earliest stages of cervical cancer is the Papanicolaou smear. A single Papanicolaou smear is about 95% effective in detecting desquamated malignant cells from the cervix and vagina. The specimens should be obtained from the posterior vaginal fornix and the external os of the cervix. The squamocolumnar junction should be adequately sampled. Any clinically suspicious lesion should be subjected to biopsy regardless of the cytologic findings, even during pregnancy.

The possibility of rendering carcinoma of the cervix a preventable disease is still far from realized because only about 10% of all women in the United States are routinely screened cytologically. These women, furthermore, often belong to groups with a low prevalence of cervical carcinoma. A larger group of women may be screened through the use of irrigation smears, which the patient obtains herself. Disadvantages of that method include greater error in collection of the specimen and the lack of a simultaneous pelvic examination.

The Papanicolaou smear may be reported by Class (I through V), by narrative description, or simply as positive, suspicious, or negative. Classes I and II show no evidence of malignant cells; Class III is suspicious; and Classes IV and V are positive for malignant cells.

Because *cytology* is only a *screening* method, no therapy is to be based on the cytologic findings alone. Instead, a suspicious or positive smear must be investigated further. *Treatment* is based only on a *histologic diagnosis*. The management of the abnormal Papanicolaou smear is diagrammed in Table 8. A suspicious smear without a clinical lesion may be repeated before histologic investigation, but a frankly positive smear should be confirmed without delay. Any *gross lesion* must be subjected at once to *biopsy*. A clinically normal cervix should be investigated by colposcopically directed biopsy (p. 129), cone biopsy (p. 130), or, less commonly today, multiple punch biopsies. Iodine-negative areas that do not contain glycogen may indicate epithelial atypia and suggest the areas for punch biopsy. The number of cone biopsies performed has been reduced by the wider use of colposcopy.

The colposcope provides a magnification of 40 times and is of aid in determining the site for biopsy. Because colposcopy cannot detect a lesion in the endocervical canal, endocervical

TABLE 8. Management of the Abnormal Papanicolaou Smear

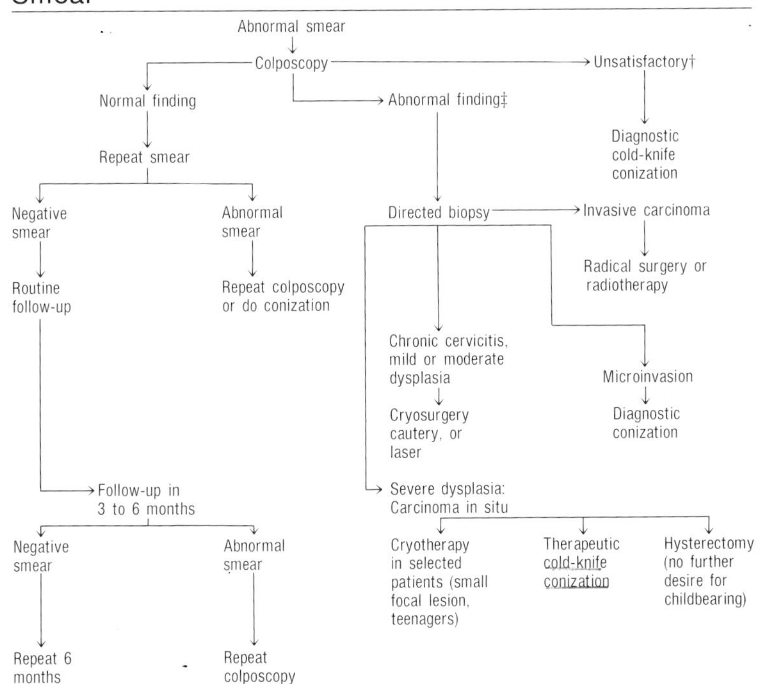

*If colposcopy is not available, conization may be required at this point.
†Satisfactory colposcopy requires that entire squamocolumnar junction be identified and entire lesion seen.
‡Biopsy is performed in presence of clinical lesion regardless of cytologic findings.

curettage or conization is required to rule out a lesion in that location. If the entire squamocolumnar junction cannot be visualized, conization is necessary to exclude invasive carcinoma. Colposcopy depends largely on the interpretation of vascular patterns. A satisfactory colposcopic examination requires complete visualization of the entire squamocolumnar junction and all suspicious lesions.

If the *punch biopsies* reveal *invasive cancer,* it is *not necessary* to perform a diagnostic *cone.* If they reveal a lesion *less extensive* than invasive cancer, a satisfactory *colposcopy* or a *cone* is *required* to rule out the coexistence of a more advanced lesion.

The complications of conization (p. 130) include bleeding, parametritis, and injury to the internal os. Where no other method of excluding invasion is available, however, the cone is still required for diagnosis and treatment.

Staging of carcinoma of the cervix is crucial for decisions about treatment and for comparison of the results of treatment in various centers.

Stage 0 is carcinoma in situ, preinvasive carcinoma, or intraepithelial carcinoma.

Stage I is invasive carcinoma confined to the cervix. (Extension to the corpus should be disregarded in staging.) *Stage Ia* is *microinvasive* carcinoma (early stromal invasion). *Stage Ib* includes all more advanced lesions.

There is still no consensus about the definition of microinvasive carcinoma of the cervix. One logical definition requires that there be not more than 3 mm of invasion below the base of the epithelium and that there be no lymphatic or hematogenous involvement or confluence of microinvasive tongues.

Occult carcinoma is a histologically invasive cancer that cannot be detected by routine clinical examination. It is classified as Stage Ib,occ. Other cases of Stage Ib carcinoma of the cervix are clinically detectable.

Stage II involves the vagina (exclusive of the lowest third), the parametria (but not to the side walls of the pelvis), or both vagina and one or both parametria.

Stage IIa lesions involve the vagina but not the parametria.

Stage IIb lesions involve the parametria with or without the vagina.

Stage IIIa lesions involve the lowest third of the vagina, and *Stage IIIb* lesions reach one or both pelvic side walls. Hydronephrosis or a nonfunctioning kidney relegates the lesion to Stage III.

Stage IV lesions involve the mucosa of the bladder or rectum (*Stage IVa*) or have distant metastases (*Stage IVb*).

Any patient with a cervical carcinoma that may require radical surgical procedures or radiotherapy should have a diagnostic investigation that includes as a minimum the following: complete blood count, chest roentgenogram, intravenous pyelogram, cystoscopy, proctoscopy, barium enema, bone scan, and hepatic and renal function tests.

Although the involvement of lymph nodes does not affect the staging of carcinoma of the cervix, it does affect the prognosis. The frequencies of involvement of the lymph nodes in the various stages of cervical carcinoma are as follows: Stage I, 15%; Stage II, 30%; Stage III, 45%; and Stage IV, 60%.

The *treatment* of carcinoma of the cervix depends on the *stage* of the lesion. Severe *dysplasias* and *carcinoma in situ* (Stage 0) may be treated with *therapeutic cone* with close *follow-up* in the woman who desires children. Other conservative treatments include *cryosurgery*, electrocautery, and possibly the CO_2 laser. In older women and multiparas the treatment of choice is *total hysterectomy* (vaginal or abdominal) with a large vaginal cuff. *Invasive cancer* is treated by *radical surgical procedures or radiation*, depending on the stage.

Surgical treatment is required for radioresistant lesions and for recurrences after full radiation. Radiation is employed in patients who present poor operative risks and for some recurrences after surgical treatment. In many cases almost identical cure rates are obtained by surgical or radiotherapeutic means.

Stage I lesions may be treated by radical hysterectomy and pelvic lymphadenectomy or by radiation. Because the likelihood of lymph node involvement in Stage Ia lesions is only about 2%, it may be safe to treat these minimally invasive lesions as though they were intraepithelial carcinomas. Some Stage IIa lesions may be treated by radical hysterectomy, but most Stage IIb lesions are better treated by radiation. Stage III lesions are treated best by radiation. Stage IV lesions are occasionally cured by ultraradical surgical procedures such as exenteration (p. 133). This drastic treatment should be employed in advanced lesions or recurrences only for cure and not for palliation.

Radiation therapy of cervical carcinoma usually involves an internal and an external source. The internal treatment typically consists of intrauterine and intravaginal radium, cesium, or other radioactive sources. ^{60}Cobalt or x-radiation is used for the external source to increase the dose to the pelvic side walls. In certain circumstances the external therapy is delivered before the intravaginal radiation.

Radiation therapy is frequently administered by afterloading techniques. Hollow applicators designed to carry a radioactive material are implanted or inserted into the area to be treated. Their position is checked before any of the radioactive material is inserted. The advantage of this technique is the minimization of exposure of the personnel to the radiation.

Understanding the principles of radiotherapy of gynecologic cancer, particularly carcinoma of the cervix, requires definition of certain terms. A curie is a special unit of radioactivity equal to 3.70×10^{10} disintegrations per second. The curie (Ci) is based on the rate of disintegration of one gram of radium. A gamma ray is a proton emitted from the nucleus of a radioactive atom, differing from an x-ray photon only with respect to origin. A roentgen (R) is a special unit of the radiation quantity "exposure," equal to an electrical charge (produced by ionization) of 2.58×10^{-4} coulomb/kg of air. A rad is a unit of the radiation quantity "absorbed dose." One rad is equal to an energy absorption of 0.01 joule/kg. The rem (Roentgen-Equivalent-Man) is a special unit of the radiation protection quantity "dose equivalent." Dose equivalent is obtained by multiplying absorbed dose by a "quality factor." When dose is expressed in rads, dose equivalent is in rems.

Point A is an imaginary point lying 2 cm lateral to the cervical canal and 2 cm above the cervical os. Point B lies 3 cm lateral to point A and is used as a means of evaluating the dosage to the pelvic wall.

Complications of radical surgical procedures include fistulas, hemorrhage, and immediate operative death. Blood volume should be measured before any radical procedures and the central venous pressure monitored during and after operation. Complications of radiation include urinary frequency (cystitis), diarrhea (frequently bloody), and bowel fistulas. Stenosis of the vagina and dyspareunia may also result.

Carcinoma of the cervix complicated by pregnancy requires special consideration. Carcinoma in situ may be managed conservatively, provided every effort has been made to rule out invasion. The pregnancy may be carried to term and the patient delivered vaginally. Definitive treatment may be performed post partum. Invasive cancer must be treated during pregnancy as in the nonpregnant state. In the first trimester the patient may be subjected to radical hysterectomy or radiation treatment (which produces abortion). In the third trimester maximal delay of a few weeks to ensure reasonable likelihood of fetal survival may be justified before cesarean section and definitive treatment are performed. In the second trimester it is usually necessary to treat the carcinoma despite the nonviability or immaturity of the fetus.

The survival in carcinoma of the cervix depends on the staging, which in turn is influenced by the success of the screening program. A successful program will result in a higher proportion of intraepithelial and early invasive lesions. The five-year prognosis by stage is as follows: Stage 0—almost 100%; Stage I—85-90% (approximately equal by radiation or radical surgery); Stage II—65-75%, and Stage III—35-40% (these stages are generally better treated by radiation); and Stage IV—approximately 5-15% (by ultraradical surgical procedures).

Myomas are the *commonest benign tumors* of the uterus. About 25% of women over the age of 30 have palpable myomas. They are found most commonly in women in their *thirties* and *forties* and are larger and more common in *black* patients. The lesion consists of interlacing bundles of *smooth muscle* with only rare mitotic figures. For this reason, the tumors should be termed myomas or *leiomyomas* rather than fibroids. Since myomas are surrounded by a *pseudocapsule* of condensed uterine tissue, unlike adenomyomas or sarcomas, they may be bloodlessly *enucleated* from the normal myometrium.

The tumors range in size from microscopic lesions to huge masses filling the abdomen. They may be located within the myometrium (*intramural*); they may protrude from the external surface of the uterus (*subserous*); or they may project into the uterine cavity (*submucous*). The subserous and submucous varieties may be *sessile* or *pedunculated*. Tumors may grow between the leaves of the broad ligament (*intraligamentous*), displacing the ureters and subjecting them to danger of injury during hysterectomy. Occasionally a myoma may detach from the uterus and obtain a new blood supply from another organ (parasitic myoma).

Large myomas frequently outgrow their blood supply and undergo *degeneration*, including hyalinization, liquefaction, calcification (detectable radiologically), formation of bone and fat, and necrosis (occasionally characterized by pain and leukocytosis). Carneous, or red, degeneration, usually occurring during pregnancy, is one of the few changes in a myoma that is associated with pain. Sarcoma occurs in only a fraction of 1% of myomas.

Myomas appear to be under estrogenic control. They are tumors of the reproductive years and may be associated with other endocrine-dependent lesions such as endometrial hyperplasia, adenomyosis, and endometriosis. They may grow during pregnancy and with use of oral contraceptives, particularly those with a high proportion of estrogen.

Myomas *do not grow after the menopause*. Tumors that appear after the menopause and all cases of *postmenopausal bleeding* must be attributed to *other causes*. The most prominent sign of myomas is *abnormal uterine bleeding*. The bleeding typically begins as *prolonged menses*, which may be sufficiently severe to cause *anemia*. Intermenstrual bleeding may occur with extensive myomas but should suggest another lesion. The abnormal bleeding may be a result of increased surface area of the endometrium or interference by the myomas with normal uterine hemostasis.

Myomas may cause dysmenorrhea and a sensation of bearing down. Only rarely, even if large, will they obstruct the urinary tract or the bowel. A myoma protruding through the cervix may cause uterine cramps. Except when complicated by torsion, infarction, and carneous degeneration, myomas usually do *not cause pain*, which should therefore be attributed to *another lesion*, usually pelvic inflammatory disease or endometriosis.

Myomas have often been implicated in infertility, although associated lesions such as pelvic inflammatory disease are more often the cause. Myomas may lead to infertility by blocking the ascent of spermatozoa, occluding the oviduct, or interfering with implantation. If a pregnancy occurs, there is a greater likelihood of prematurity, abnormal presentations, dystocia, dysfunctional labor, and postpartum hemorrhage.

Diagnosis of myomas is made by *history*, an irregular, firm, *nodular uterus* on pelvic examination, and if necessary a *hysterosalpingogram* to demonstrate a filling defect (submucous myomas). Differential diagnosis includes *pregnancy*, *ovarian tumors*, and *uterine anomalies*. The pregnant uterus is usually softer and more symmetric, and the chorionic gonadotropin test is positive. It is impossible on physical examination to distinguish myomas from ovarian tumors with certainty after the aggregate pelvic mass has reached *12 weeks' gestational size*. By that time the tumor has risen above the pelvic brim and the ovaries can no longer be palpated separately.

It is most important that the *cause of bleeding* in a patient with myomas be *ascertained before hysterectomy*. Bleeding in a patient with myomas does not necessarily stem from the myomas. It may be the result of a less serious lesion, such as an endometrial polyp, or a more serious disease such as carcinoma of the cervix or corpus. A *Papanicolaou smear* and a *fractional curettage* should therefore precede definitive therapy of myomas.

Management of myomas may be *conservative* or may entail *myomectomy* or *hysterectomy. No treatment* is required in a woman of reproductive age if the tumors do not cause bleeding, pain, or infertility, and if they are less than 12 weeks' gestational size. In a patient near the menopause, conservative therapy may be employed after a curettage has ruled out a malignant lesion. *Postmenopausal bleeding* requires *immediate diagnosis* and treatment.

The usual treatment of *symptomatic myomas* is *hysterectomy.* Myomectomy is logically performed only in a woman of reproductive age who desires children and in whom there is no other factor preventing pregnancy. *Laparotomy* is indicated for any mass greater than 12 weeks' size to *rule out an ovarian tumor.* A smaller mass in a patient near the menopause may be managed conservatively if asymptomatic. Rapid growth in the absence of pregnancy or oral contraceptives requires investigation.

A small uterus may be removed by the vaginal route, but large myomas are best removed by *total abdominal hysterectomy.* The decision to remove the ovaries is based on their condition and the patient's age.

Endometrial polyps are finger-like projections of the endometrium into the uterine cavity. They consist of glands and stroma and vary from microscopic size to several centimeters in length. In only a small percentage of cases does malignant change occur. Polyps are found in all age groups, but mostly in older women. They present with *metrorrhagia* or *postmenopausal bleeding*. Diagnosis is made by *fractional curettage,* which may also be *therapeutic.* The differential diagnosis includes endocervical polyps, myomas, and carcinomas of the cervix and endometrium.

A placental polyp may occasionally simulate the more common endometrial polyp. It is a cause of delayed postpartum bleeding.

Hyperplasia of the endometrium is usually considered to be related to *unopposed estrogen.* The *cystic and glandular* (Swiss cheese) variety is *not* considered a *premalignant* lesion. *Adenomatous hyperplasia* is more serious. *Atypical* adenomatous hyperplasia is often a *precursor of carcinoma* of the endometrium. Both diagnosis and treatment may often be achieved through curettage. *Recurrent* adenomatous hyperplasia in the perimenopausal or postmenopausal woman is best treated by *hysterectomy*.

Carcinoma of the corpus accounts for about 20% of all gynecologic cancers. In recent years it has become more prevalent in relation to carcinoma of the cervix. It affects predominantly *menopausal* and *postmenopausal* women. Its peak incidence is at age 55, or 10 years later than that of carcinoma of the cervix. In white patients of low parity and high socioeconomic status, the ratio of incidence of carcinoma of the cervix to that of carcinoma of the corpus may be 1:1, whereas in black patients of low socioeconomic status and high parity, the ratio of cancer of the cervix to cancer of the corpus may be as high as 10:1.

Although there is abundant evidence to support the relation of *unopposed estrogen* and *anovulation* to carcinoma of the corpus, there is no unanimity that the estrogen per se is the carcinogen. The risk of carcinoma of the corpus in *postmenopausal women* receiving *replacement therapy* with estrogens is increased between threefold and eightfold (p. 218). Carcinoma of the corpus is more commonly found in the *obese nullipara* and the patient with a *late menopause and poor fertility*. *Hypertension, diabetes,* and cardiovascular disease are often associated.

Cancers of the endometrium are usually *adenocarcinomas*. The *in-situ form* may be indistinguishable from severe atypical adenomatous hyperplasia. The glands are crowded back to back, with individual cells exhibiting the criteria of malignancy.

About 15% of carcinomas of the endometrium have squamous metaplasia (adenoacanthoma). This lesion does not differ significantly from ordinary adenocarcinoma with respect to therapy and prognosis.

Carcinoma of the endometrium remains *localized* in the uterus for a long while and then may *spread widely* by the *vascular* route. Extension may occur also along the peritoneum or by penetration of the myometrium. Pyometra is an occasional complication. About 10% metastasize early to the ovary. When spread occurs to the cervix, the behavior and treatment of the tumor resemble those of carcinoma of the cervix. Prognosis of endometrial carcinoma is adversely affected by poor differentiation of the tumor and deep myometrial invasion.

The main sign of carcinoma of the corpus is *metrorrhagia*. Older women usually present with *postmenopausal bleeding*. In some series about one third of all cases of postmenopausal bleeding are caused by carcinoma of the corpus.

The *Papanicolaou smear* is *less reliable* for diagnosis in this disease than in carcinoma of the cervix. Results may be improved by several techniques that sample the endometrium directly, such as the jet wash, but the mainstay of diagnosis is *curettage*. A *fractional curettage* is required to distinguish adenocarcinoma of the corpus from that of the cervix. A hysterosalpingogram should not be performed in the presence of suspected carcinoma of the corpus.

Stage 0 is carcinoma in situ.

Stage I carcinoma of the endometrium is confined to the corpus. In Stage Ia the length of the uterine cavity is 8 cm or less, whereas in Stage Ib the length is more than 8 cm. Stage Ia is also subdivided according to the histologic type of the adenocarcinoma. G_1 is a highly differentiated adenocarcinoma; G_2 is a differentiated adenocarcinoma with partly solid areas; and G_3 is a predominantly solid or entirely undifferentiated carcinoma. Stage II extends to the cervix. Stage III carcinoma of the corpus has spread beyond the uterus but not outside the true pelvis. In Stage IV the tumor has spread beyond the confines of the pelvis or has involved the mucosa of the bladder or rectum.

The mainstay of *treatment* in carcinoma of the corpus is surgical, that is, *total abdominal hysterectomy and bilateral salpingo-oophorectomy*. Conventional treatment involves the intracavitary application of *radium* or another radioactive source four to six weeks before hysterectomy to destroy the superficial tumor and to decrease the likelihood of metastases, particularly to the vaginal vault.

Some gynecologists perform the hysterectomy without the delay of four to six weeks, and others are eliminating radiation entirely, particularly in cases of small uteri and well-differentiated tumors. Stage II lesions are usually treated by full radiation, as in carcinoma of the cervix, perhaps with the addition of simple total hysterectomy and bilateral salpingo-oophorectomy. In Stages III and IV the results of both radiation and surgical treatment are poor. High doses of progestins have been used for palliation and temporary control of recurrent or metastatic lesions.

The prognosis of early, well-differentiated Stage I lesions should be close to 100%; the prognosis for all Stage I lesions is about 80%. In Stage II the cure rate drops to about 30%. In Stage III it is less than 20%, and in Stage IV it is less than 5%. The total five-year survival in carcinoma of the corpus is slightly over 50%.

Sarcoma of the corpus is much less common than carcinoma of the endometrium in this country. Leiomyosarcoma is the commonest of the pure homologous sarcomas. It may arise from the normal myometrium or from a myoma. It presents with bleeding and vaginal discharge and may be suspected when an apparent myoma grows rapidly. The treatment is total abdominal hysterectomy and bilateral salpingo-oophorectomy. The additional benefit of radiation is questionable.

Sarcomas may also arise from the endometrial stroma. These tumors, as well as mixed mesodermal malignant lesions (which are currently being reported in greater numbers), are treated by total abdominal hysterectomy and bilateral salpingo-oophorectomy. The effect of radiation is small and the prognosis is generally poor.

Benign neoplasms of the fallopian tube include myomas, hemangiomas, and fibromas, all very uncommon lesions. The more common parovarian cysts, such as the hydatid of Morgagni, are of little clinical significance. Many of these structures, formerly considered to be of mesonephric origin, are now believed to be paramesonephric.

The fallopian tube is the least common site of carcinoma of the female genitalia. On physical examination tubal neoplasms are usually confused with ovarian masses. Histologically, cancer of the oviduct is usually an adenocarcinoma, which spreads locally and by lymphatics. The lesion may present with vaginal bleeding, lower abdominal pain, and watery vaginal discharge (hydrorrhea). It should be suspected when curettings are negative in women with postmenopausal bleeding, particularly if there is an adnexal mass. The lesion is often found accidentally at laparotomy. Treatment is total abdominal hysterectomy and bilateral salpingo-oophorectomy. Carcinoma in the fallopian tube is more often metastatic, usually from the ovary or corpus.

All *adnexal masses* must be considered potential *ovarian tumors* until proved otherwise. Of all ovarian tumors about 30 to 40% are *malignant.* As the detection and treatment of early carcinomas of the cervix and corpus improve, carcinoma of the *ovary* becomes *increasingly important.* In some series, the ovary is the most common site of gynecologic cancer, but in general ovarian carcinoma accounts for between 10 and 20% of all female genital cancers. Ovarian cancer affects *all age groups,* with the greatest frequency in the 50- to 60-year group.

The ovary is unusual in that it is a common site of both *primary* and *metastatic* lesions. The *poor prognosis* is related to several factors: there is *no detectable in-situ form of* ovarian cancer; *spread* occurs *rapidly* by *peritoneal implantation* as well as *vascular* channels; and there are *no early signs* and *symptoms.* Routine vaginal cytology has not been effective in detecting preclinical ovarian carcinoma.

The *clinical manifestations* of ovarian cancer suggest an *advanced lesion.* They include abdominal pain, increase in abdominal girth, palpable abdominal and pelvic masses, gastrointestinal and urinary tract complaints, ascites, and thrombophlebitis. *Nonspecific* lower abdominal *complaints* and dysmenorrhea are more common than irregular vaginal bleeding. Anorexia and cachexia occur still later. Any ovarian tumor may cause an *acute surgical emergency* by undergoing an accident such as rupture, torsion, hemorrhage, infection, infarction, and incarceration.

Differential diagnosis includes carcinoma of the rectum or sigmoid, diverticulosis, retroperitoneal tumors, ectopic pregnancy, pelvic kidney, endometriosis, pelvic inflammatory disease, and pregnancy. The lesion with which a solid tumor of the ovary is most commonly confused is a *uterine myoma*. An ovarian cyst may be differentiated from *ascites* by physical findings (p. 14).

Detection of of an ovarian tumor is followed by *laparotomy* without delay except in special circumstances: in a woman in the *reproductive* years, a *cystic unilateral mass less than 5 cm* in diameter may be managed conservatively because it may well be a functional cyst of the ovary. Proper management in such cases involves reexamination of the patient in about six weeks. Ovulation should be suppressed by oral contraceptives during the period of observation to avoid confusion resulting from the formation of a new functional cyst. If the mass has *regressed, no further treatment* is required. If it has remained stationary or enlarged, laparotomy is indicated. In all other cases immediate *laparotomy* is required for ovarian tumors, including all *solid* or *bilateral* masses and all tumors greater than 5 to 6 cm in diameter. A palpable ovary in a postmenopausal woman should be regarded as a possible malignant tumor.

Diagnostic measures before laparotomy often include intravenous pyelography, proctoscopy, and upper or lower gastrointestinal roentgenograms, depending on the symptoms and signs. A *scout film* of the abdomen may identify the opacity characteristic of a *benign cystic teratoma* or may visualize a tooth or piece of bone.

Staging of ovarian carcinoma is done at the time of laparotomy. Because of the enormous variety of histologic types and the individualization of management required, operations on patients with suspected carcinoma of the ovary should be performed only by the gynecologist who is thoroughly familiar with the surgical pathology. The laparotomy should include inspection of the undersurface of the diaphragm and the retroperitoneal lymph nodes, with biopsy of suspicious lesions.

Staging of ovarian carcinoma is based on findings at clinical examination and surgical exploration. Stage I carcinoma is limited to the ovaries. Stage Ia is limited to one ovary, without ascites. In Stage Ia_1 there is no tumor on the external surface and the capsule is intact; in Stage Ia_2 there is tumor on the external surface, a ruptured capsule, or both. Stage Ib involves both ovaries, without ascites. In Stage Ib_1 there is no tumor on the external surface and the capsule is intact; in Stage Ib_2 there is tumor on the external surface, a ruptured capsule, or both. In Stage Ic one or both ovaries are involved, with ascites or malignant cells in the peritoneal fluid.

Stage II carcinoma of the ovary involves one or both ovaries with spread elsewhere in the pelvis, with or without ascites. Stage IIa has spread to the uterus, oviducts, or both; Stage IIb involves other pelvic organs. A tumor in Stage II complicated by ascites or positive peritoneal washings is relegated to Stage IIc.

In Stage III the growth involves one or both ovaries with intraperitoneal metastases outside the pelvis, positive retroperitoneal nodes, or both. Tumor limited to the pelvis with histologically proven malignant extension to small bowel or omentum is classified as Stage III.

In Stage IV the cancer involves one or both ovaries with distant metastases. If pleural effusion is present, malignant cells must be found in the fluid to justify the classification of Stage IV. Metastases in the hepatic parenchyma are considered evidence of Stage IV.

Enucleation of the tumor or *unilateral oophorectomy* is acceptable treatment only for *well-encapsulated benign tumors in young women*. The basic surgical treatment for *malignant tumors* of the ovary is total abdominal *hysterectomy with bilateral salpingo-oophorectomy*. Excision of accessible masses of tumor (debulking) and the *omentum* (to remove microscopic metastases) are justified, but ultraradical procedures (exenteration) are not indicated. Occasionally, *postoperative radiation* may be used to treat a technically inoperable lesion. This radiation may shrink the tumor sufficiently to allow a *second*, more successful, *operation*. Most ovarian tumors are *not radiosensitive*, however, and can only be palliated temporarily by radiotherapy.

Chemotherapy has been used successfully for palliation of persistent or recurrent ovarian cancer. Its effectiveness depends on the volume of residual tumor after surgical resection, the histologic type and grade of the tumor, and the original stage of the disease. A *second laparotomy* with biopsy of suspicious areas should be performed before discontinuing chemotherapy.

Combined chemotherapy involves use of several classes of drugs, including alkylating agents such as chlorambucil, antimetabolites such as methotrexate, and antibiotics such as actinomycin D. Although these drugs may prolong life, serious side effects may occur, including leukopenia and gastrointestinal disturbances. During chemotherapy the leukocyte and platelet counts must be carefully monitored. Management of incurable cancer of the ovary includes antibiotics for urinary tract infections, paracentesis for relief of ascites, and narcotics for pain in the terminal stages.

The five-year cure rate in ovarian cancer is still only about 20 to 30% because 50 to 80% of the tumors have spread beyond the ovary at the time of laparotomy. The survival drops from about 65% in Stage I to less than 40% in Stage II, and only about 5% in Stages III and IV. The histologic type is an important determinant of the prognosis. In general, the more poorly differentiated the lesion, the worse is the prognosis. Mucinous and endometrioid carcinomas, for example, have a generally better prognosis than do serous carcinomas.

Although it is virtually impossible to construct a classification of ovarian tumors that satisfies all gynecologists and pathologists, the scheme shown in Table 9, which lists only the most common tumors, has the advantage of simplicity. A more detailed classification appears on pages 185–188.

Follicle cysts of the ovary signify failure of ovulation and may be a cause of *dysfunctional uterine bleeding*. They do not exceed 6 cm in diameter and regress in one or two months. The polycystic ovary associated with the Stein-Leventhal syndrome is discussed on page 211.

A *corpus luteum cyst* is lined by luteinized granulosa cells, which secrete progesterone. Since the associated clinical features include delay of menses and a unilateral adnexal mass, the lesion is often confused with *ectopic pregnancy* (p. 80).

Theca lutein cysts form in response to high levels of chorionic gonadotropin. They are commonly associated with trophoblastic growths (p. 82), but are occasionally found with normal pregnancy. They regress after the gonadotropic stimulus is removed and should not be excised surgically. Endometrial

TABLE 9. Simplified Classification of Common Ovarian Tumors

I. Nonneoplastic (functional, physiologic) Ovarian Cysts

- A. *Follicle cyst*
- B. *Corpus luteum and theca lutein cysts*
- C. *Endometrial cysts*

II. True Neoplasms

- A. *Benign*
  1. Cystic
     - a. Serous
     - b. Mucinous
     - c. Teratoma (dermoid cyst)
  2. Solid
     - a. Fibroma
     - b. Brenner tumor
  3. Hormonally active*
     - a. Granulosa-theca tumors (estrogen-producing)
     - b. Arrhenoblastoma (androgen-producing)
- B. *Malignant*
  1. Primary
     - a. Adenocarcinoma
     - b. Serous cystadenocarcinoma
     - c. Mucinous cystadenocarcinoma
     - d. Endometrial adenocarcinoma
     - e. Solid teratoma
     - f. Dysgerminoma†
  2. Metastatic

*These tumors are often considered to be of low-grade malignancy
†This tumor is often of low-grade malignancy

cysts, a manifestation of endometriosis (p. 155), are also classified as nonneoplastic cysts. Because they often contain old blood they are a common variety of "chocolate cyst."

Parovarian cysts rarely reach large size. When palpable, they are often misdiagnosed as ovarian cysts.

The recent World Health Organization classification of ovarian tumors is shown in Table 10.

TABLE 10. W.H.O. Classification of Ovarian Tumors

I. Common Epithelial Tumors

A. *Serous tumors*

1. Benign
   a. cystadenoma and papillary cystadenoma
   b. surface papilloma
   c. adenofibroma and cystadenofibroma
2. Borderline malignancy (carcinomas of low malignant potential)
   a. cystadenoma and papillary cystadenoma
   b. surface papilloma
   c. adenofibroma and cystadenofibroma
3. Malignant
   a. adenocarcinoma, papillary adenocarcinoma, and papillary cystadenocarcinoma
   b. surface papillary carcinoma
   c. Malignant adenofibroma and cystadenofibroma

B. *Mucinous tumors*

1. Benign
   a. cystadenoma
   b. adenofibroma and cystadenofibroma
2. Borderline malignancy (carcinomas of low malignant potential)
   a. cystadenoma
   b. adenofibroma and cystadenofibroma
3. Malignant
   a. adenocarcinoma and cystadenocarcinoma
   b. malignant adenofibroma and cystadenofibroma

C. *Endometrioid tumors*

1. Benign
   a. adenoma and cystadenoma
   b. adenofibroma and cystadenofibroma
2. Borderline malignancy (carcinomas of low malignant potential
   a. adenoma and cystadenoma
   b. adenofibroma and cystadenofibroma
3. Malignant
   a. carcinoma

TABLE 10 (*Continued*)

- i. adenocarcinoma
- ii. adenoacanthoma
- iii. malignant adenofibroma and cystadenofibroma
- b. endometrioid stromal sarcomas
- c. mesodermal (müllerian) mixed tumors, homologous and heterologous

D. *Clear cell (mesonephroid) tumors*

1. Benign: adenofibroma
2. Borderline malignancy (carcinomas of low malignant potential)
3. Malignant: carcinoma and adenocarcinoma

E. *Brenner tumors*

1. Benign
2. Borderline malignancy (proliferating)
3. Malignant

F. *Mixed epithelial tumors*

1. Benign
2. Borderline malignancy
3. Malignant

G. *Unclassified carcinoma*

H. *Unclassified epithelial tumors*

II. Sex Cord Stromal Tumors

A. *Granulosa-stromal cell tumors*

1. Granulosa cell tumor
2. Tumors in the thecoma-fibroma group
   - a. thecoma
   - b. fibroma
   - c. unclassified

B. *Androblastomas; Sertoli-Leydig cell tumors*

1. Well differentiated
   - a. tubular androblastoma; Sertoli cell tumor (tubular adenoma of Pick)

TABLE 10 (*Continued*)

b. tubular androblastoma with lipid storage; Sertoli cell tumor with lipid storage (folliculome lipidique)
c. Sertoli-Leydig cell tumor (tubular adenoma with Leydig cells)
d. Leydig cell tumor; hilus cell tumor

2. Intermediate differentiation
3. Poorly differentiated (sarcomatoid)
4. With heterologous elements

C. *Gynandroblastoma*
D. *Unclassified*

III. Lipid (Lipoid) Cell Tumors

IV. Germ Cell Tumors

A. *Dysgerminoma*
B. *Endodermal sinus tumor*
C. *Embryonal carcinoma*
D. *Polyembryoma*
E. *Choriocarcinoma*
F. *Teratomas*

1. Immature
2. Mature
   a. solid
   b. cystic
      i. dermoid cyst (mature cystic teratoma)
      ii. dermoid cyst with malignant transformation
3. Monodermal and highly specialized
   a. struma ovarii
   b. carcinoid
   c. struma ovarii and carcinoid
   d. others

G. *Mixed forms*

V. Gonadoblastoma

A. *Pure*
B. *Mixed with dysgerminoma or other form of germ cell tumor*

TABLE 10 (*Continued*)

VI. Soft Tissue Tumors Not Specific to Ovary

VII. Unclassified Tumors

VIII. Secondary (Metastatic) Tumors

IX. Tumor-like Conditions

A. *Pregnancy luteoma*
B. *Hyperplasia of ovarian stroma and hyperthecosis*
C. *Massive edema*
D. *Solitary follicle cyst and corpus luteum cyst*
E. *Multiple follicle cysts (polycystic ovaries)*
F. *Multiple luteinized follicle cysts, corpora lutea, or both*
G. *Endometriosis*
H. *Surface-epithelial inclusion cysts (germinal inclusion cysts)*
I. *Simple cysts*
J. *Inflammatory lesions*
K. *Parovarian cysts*

Serous cystadenoma is the *most common true neoplasm* of the ovary, accounting for 20 to 25% of all ovarian tumors. It is commonly multicystic and is bilateral in 20% or more of cases. It occurs in the reproductive and postmenopausal age groups. Histologically the epithelial lining resembles that of the fallopian tube, and calcareous concretions called psammoma bodies may be found. As may all pedunculated tumors, the serous cystadenoma may undergo torsion. The *papillary variety* is more likely to undergo malignant change. About 25% of the papillary serous cystadenomas are *potentially or actually malignant.* Bilateral tumors and those in which the capsule has been penetrated are more likely to be malignant.

The *mucinous cystadenoma* accounts for about 10% of all ovarian tumors. It is often multilocular, and about 5% are bilateral. The likelihood of malignant change is about 5 to 10%. The epithelial lining of the cyst resembles that of the endocervix or the small intestine. These tumors may attain very large size.

Rupture of the cyst may produce the condition known as pseudomyxoma peritonei, which may be fatal.

The benign cystic teratoma (dermoid cyst) is the second most common benign ovarian tumor, accounting for about 15% of all ovarian tumors. It contains derivatives of all three germ layers, although skin and its appendages predominate. The tissues found in the benign teratoma are *mature* and well differentiated. They commonly occur in the third decade of life. About 25% of dermoid cysts are bilateral. Rupture of this tumor may produce a severe *chemical peritonitis*. Diagnosis of a dermoid cyst may occasionally be made preoperatively by roentgenologic demonstration of teeth or bone.

A special variety of dermoid, in which thyroid tissue predominates, is the struma ovarii. This tumor may produce hyperthyroidism, which regresses after removal of the neoplasm. The risk of malignant change in a benign cystic teratoma is only about 1%. The most commonly associated cancer is squamous cell carcinoma.

The most *common benign solid tumor* of the ovary is the *fibroma*. This neoplasm accounts for about 5% of all ovarian tumors. About 90% are unilateral, and they occur more commonly after the menopause. There is less than a 1% likelihood of malignant transformation. In about 25% of cases the tumor is complicated by *ascites* and *hydrothorax* (Meigs' syndrome). The *effusions regress* after removal of the tumor. The cause of the hydrothorax and ascites is not clear.

The Brenner tumor, which is usually unilateral, accounts for about 1 to 2% of all ovarian tumors. It is a solid benign neoplasm with a very small likelihood of malignant change. It is usually found in women above the age of 40. Histologically it consists of a fibrous stroma surrounding epithelioid cells with longitudinally grooved nuclei.

Endocrinologically active tumors of the ovary are difficult to classify. They are generally of a *low degree of malignancy* and are therefore often considered with both the benign and the malignant tumors. They may be classified according to *histo-*

logic type or *endocrine* effects. The interconvertibility of the steroid hormones adds to the difficulty in classification. These tumors as a group are often described as *gonadal stromal tumors* or mesenchymomas. In the *granulosa-theca cell tumors,* one or the other element may predominate or occur exclusively. In general, these are *estrogen-producing* lesions, which account for about 10% of all solid ovarian tumors.

The *granulosa cell tumor* accounts for between 1 and 3% of all ovarian tumors. About 95% are unilateral, and all are generally small. Histologically the granulosa cells form a columnar or folliculoid pattern. The poorly differentiated tumors may appear sarcomatoid. Granulosa cell tumors may cause *precocious puberty* in the child or *postmenopausal bleeding* in the older patient. In a woman in the reproductive years they are likely to cause *abnormal uterine bleeding* or *endometrial hyperplasia.* About 10 to 30% undergo *malignant change.* In the *young patient, unilateral oophorectomy* may be attempted, but in the *older patient* the treatment of choice is total abdominal *hysterectomy with bilateral salpingo-oophorectomy.*

Thecomas are also *estrogen-producing* tumors of the ovary. They too account for a small percentage of all ovarian tumors. In general, they are small and unilateral. Not more than 1% of these tumors have malignant potential. The tumors histologically resemble fibromas, from which they may be distinguished by appropriate lipid stains. Luteinization of an estrogen-producing tumor may be associated with a progestational endometrium. According to some investigators, there is an increased risk of endometrial carcinoma in patients with these tumors. Treatment of thecomas is based on the same principles as that of granulosa cell tumors.

A typical masculinizing tumor of the ovary is the arrhenoblastoma. About 95% of these uncommon tumors are unilateral, and the majority occur in women under the age of 35. The malignant potential is about 20 to 25%. A well-differentiated form of the tumor is the Pick, or testicular, adenoma. The Leydig cells, which are the source of androgen, are not prominent in the highly differentiated testicular adenoma. Treatment is usually total abdominal hysterectomy and bilateral salpingo-oophorectomy. Defeminization is followed by masculinization, or virilization. The normal sequence is amenorrhea, involution of the breasts and uterus, and infertility, followed by hirsutism, acne, deepening of the voice, and hypertrophy of the clitoris.

Still less common masculinizing tumors of the ovary are the hilus cell and the adrenal rest tumors. The hilus cell tumor has about a 1% malignant potential. Microscopically, the hilus cells resemble Leydig cells and may contain crystalloids of Reinke.

Primary adenocarcinoma of the ovary is basically a solid tumor, which may contain cystic or necrotic areas. It is *relatively undifferentiated,* commonly *bilateral,* and *highly malignant.* Since the tumor spreads rapidly by seeding of the peritoneum and omentum, the patient with this lesion often presents with *ascites.*

Serous cystadenocarcinoma is the *most common cancer* of the ovary, accounting for about half of all ovarian carcinomas. In more than 50% of cases, it presents as *bilateral cystic* or loculated ovarian masses with ascites. The *papillary projections* may detach and implant widely in the peritoneal cavity.

Mucinous cystadenocarcinoma accounts for about 10 to 15% of all ovarian cancers. The tumors are often large and multilocular, with numerous areas of hemorrhage. About 25% are bilateral.

The cure rate of *endometrial adenocarcinoma of the ovary* is better than that of the other cystic ovarian cancers.

Solid teratomas of the ovary usually contain poorly differentiated derivatives of all three germ layers. They are found more commonly in the young patient. The degree of malignancy is high and the prognosis is poor.

The *dysgerminoma* arises from the undifferentiated germ cell and is histologically identical with the *seminoma* of the testis. The tumor is found in young adults, about 75% occurring before the age of 26. The dysgerminoma is bilateral in 10 to 20% of cases. Microscopically, it consists of large ovoid cells separated by delicate septa of connective tissue with a sprinkling of leukocytes. The degree of *malignancy* is *variable.* Bilateral tumors and those in which the capsule has been broken have a poorer prognosis. The tumor occasionally produces chorionic gonadotropin (with or without associated teratoid trophoblast) and is sometimes found in intersexes. The usual treatment in the patient who has completed her family is *total abdominal hysterectomy and bilateral salpingo-oophorectomy.* Occasionally in the *young patient,* a *well-encapsulated unilateral* tumor may be treated by *unilateral oophorectomy.* This tumor, unlike most ovarian neoplasms, is rather *radiosensitive.*

About 20 to 25% of all ovarian tumors are metastatic. Common primary sites are the *endometrium,* the *gastrointestinal tract,* and the *breast.* A Krukenberg tumor is usually metastatic from the gastrointestinal tract. Microscopically, it consists of signet-ring (fat-containing) cells in a dense fibrous stroma.

UNIT VI

Gynecologic Endocrinology and Related Topics

Basic understanding of gynecologic endocrine syndromes requires knowledge of general endocrinology, for lesions of the *central nervous system, hypothalamus, pituitary,* and *other endocrine glands* directly affect the function of the *ovary* and *uterus.* Furthermore, reproductive endocrine function is affected by *metabolic* disorders, *systemic* diseases, and *psychogenic* factors. The information in this Unit is helpful in understanding further the physiologic changes in *pregnancy* (p. 24) and the mode of action and side effects of steroidal *contraceptives* (p. 231).

The most common endocrine syndromes involve a *delay* in *menarche* or *puberty; amenorrhea* (primary or secondary); *defeminization, virilization,* and *hirsutism;* and *ambiguous genitalia,* or *intersexuality.* In addition, management of the *menopause* and *infertility* often include endocrinologic diagnosis and therapy. Except for the most obvious endocrinopathies, these patients should be *referred to a specialist* in gynecologic endocrinology for diagnosis and therapy.

Abnormal uterine bleeding frequently results from endocrine dysfunction, but it is mandatory to rule out all other causes, especially neoplasms, before instituting hormonal therapy.

Dysmenorrhea and *premenstrual tension* are common problems that may have an endocrine component.

Finally, a knowledge of normal endocrine function is requisite to a rational discussion of *human sexuality* (Unit VIII).

■ Puberty

Puberty is the period when a person becomes *sexually mature,* the reproductive organs become functional, and the secondary sexual characteristics become developed. Its onset varies somewhat with racial, hereditary, social, and nutritional factors. *Menarche,* or the onset of menses, occurs about two years after the onset of puberty, which normally lasts between four and eight years. Puberty begins about two years earlier in girls than in boys. Menarche normally occurs between 10 and 16 years of age, with an average of 12.5 years in North America. The age of menarche has gradually fallen during the last few decades. Since the first few cycles are usually *anovulatory,* fertility is ordinarily not established until about two years after menarche. The changes accompanying puberty normally occur in a well-defined sequence: development of the *breasts* (*thelarche*), growth of *pubic hair* (*adrenarche*), growth of axillary hair, and finally *menses*.

The first sign of puberty is usually the appearance of downy pubic hair. A small growth spurt in height and weight is then followed by elevation of the nipples and the growth of coarse and curly pubic hair. Budding of the breasts and enlargement of the areolae precede the marked growth spurt. Enlargement of the labia, further growth of pubic hair, and filling out of the breasts accompany the development of axillary hair. Menarche then occurs, followed by further growth of the labia and a decrease in the rate of general growth. The distribution of pubic hair is now of the adult type. Axillary hair is more abundant and the breasts approach the adult configuration. Labia are now of the adult type, annual growth decreases, and menstruation is well established.

The growth spurt in puberal girls reaches a peak about two months before menarche, or at 12.3 years of age. The growth rate then declines and ceases about 2.5 years after menarche. The epiphyses close at 16 to 17 years of age.

Precocious puberty is defined as puberty before the age of eight in girls (or 10 in boys). It is more common in girls. Another definition is menarche before the age of 10 and adrenarche before the age of 9 in girls. *Heterosexual precocity* in girls implies *virilization*. It may result from functioning tumors of the gonad, hyperplasia or neoplasia of the adrenal, or exogenous sex hormones. *Isosexual precocity* in girls implies early maturation in the female direction. It may be caused by premature stimulation of the gonads by gonadotropins, autonomous release of sex steroids by the gonad or adrenal cortex, or unusual sensitivity of sexual tissues to normal hormonal levels.

The most common form of precocious puberty is *idiopathic*, or constitutional. Other causes are tumors and other lesions of the *brain*, *exogenous estrogens*, *adrenal or ovarian tumors*, and *Albright's syndrome*.

True precocity results from a disturbance in the central nervous system. It may be accompanied by an increase in gonadotropins and ovarian estrogens, and even pregnancy.

Albright's syndrome is rare. Some authorities consider it to be primarily a disorder of the central nervous system. It comprises dysplasia of bone, brown pigmented areas of skin, and sexual and somatic precocity in girls.

In pseudopuberal precocity (precocious pseudopuberty) maturation of the sexual organs occurs without ovulation or formation of a corpus luteum. This syndrome may result from tumors of the ovary or adrenal.

In all forms of sexual precocity the patients *initially* will be *tall* for their age but because their epiphyses close prematurely, they will *ultimately* be *shorter* than average for their age. In the *true idiopathic syndrome,* gonadotropins, 17-ketosteroids, gonadal steroids, and pregnanediol are *within normal adult limits.* The *electroencephalogram* is often abnormal, however. In the *pseudosyndrome,* estrogen or testosterone is high in the absence of elevated gonadotropins.

Diagnosis requires expert evaluation. Techniques employed to rule out organic lesions of the *nervous system, gonad,* and *adrenal* include electroencephalography, cerebral angiography, and roentgenograms of the skull, in addition to complete neurologic and ophthalmologic examinations. Abdominal and pelvic lesions should be excluded by examination under anesthesia, laparoscopy, and pneumoperitoneum. Gonadotropins and gonadal hormones should be measured to distinguish true precocity from pseudoprecocity. An endometrial biopsy provides further diagnostic information.

Treatment of precocious puberty depends on the cause. *True precocity* without an organic lesion requires no direct treatment, but *pregnancy* must be *prevented* if the patient is ovulating. *Counseling* is helpful to aid the girl in her psychosexual adjustment. In the *pseudosyndrome,* treatment may be directed toward *removing the tumor* or *suppressing the hyperplastic adrenal cortex* (p. 208).

Retarded puberty may arise from dysfunction of the ovary or central nervous system. It should be evaluated by the age of 15.

Gonadal dysgenesis (p. 205), testicular feminization (p. 206), and diencephalic lesions must be excluded. The associated emaciation or obesity should be corrected.

Amenorrhea

Of all the stigmata of endocrine disorders, *amenorrhea* results from the greatest diversity of causes. It figures prominently in the differential diagnosis of *defeminization, intersexuality,* and *infertility.* An entirely satisfactory simple classification of the amenorrheas is therefore almost impossible to construct since the various etiologic subgroups are often interrelated. Investigation and treatment of amenorrhea require basic knowledge of *developmental and chromosomal abnormalities* and *general endocrinology.*

Primary amenorrhea is lack of menarche by the age of 18. Amenorrhea should be investigated by the age of 16, and preferably earlier. *Secondary amenorrhea* is the cessation of menstruation for at least three months in a woman who has had her menarche.

The causes of amenorrhea may be considered *physiologic* or *pathologic.* Amenorrhea is *normal* (physiologic) in *childhood, pregnancy, lactation,* and the *menopause.* By far the commonest cause of amenorrhea in a woman in the reproductive years is pregnancy. Amenorrhea may persist normally from six weeks to six months after pregnancy and may be prolonged somewhat by breastfeeding or stimulation of the nipples. Amenorrhea lasting longer than six months post partum may represent a pathologic *lactation amenorrhea* (p. 209).

Pathologic amenorrhea may stem from *anatomic, congenital,* or *chromosomal defects* or may reflect *dysfunction* of the *central nervous system, hypothalamus, pituitary, ovary,* or *uterus.* It may also follow in the wake of *systemic diseases, dysfunction* of the other *endocrine glands,* or *psychogenic factors* (Table 11). Before a diagnosis of amenorrhea is undertaken, *pregnancy* must be *excluded.* When the cause of amenorrhea cannot be ascertained, the disorder is often termed *idiopathic* (Table 12).

TABLE 11. Etiology of Amenorrhea

I. Physiologic
   A. *Prepuberal state*
   B. *Pregnancy*
   C. *Postpartum lactation*
   D. *Menopause*

II. Congenital Anatomic
   A. *Imperforate hymen*
   B. *Developmental anomalies*

III. Chromosomal and Genetic
   A. *Gonadal dysgenesis*
   B. *Testicular feminization*
   C. *True hermaphroditism*
   D. *Other forms of pseudohermaphroditism and intersexuality*

IV. Central Nervous System—Hypothalamic—Pituitary
   A. *Tumors and other organic lesions*
   B. *Amenorrhea-galactorrhea syndromes*
   C. *Hypogonadotropic hypogonadism*
   D. *Pituitary insufficiency*
   E. *Polycystic ovary syndrome and its variants* (*Stein-Leventhal syndrome*)
   F. *Post-pill amenorrhea* (*pituitary oversuppression*)

V. Psychogenic
   A. *Psychosis*
   B. *Emotional shock*
   C. *Pseudocyesis*
   D. *Anorexia nervosa*

VI. Systemic
   A. *Chronic disease*
   B. *Nutritional disorders*

TABLE 11. (*Continued*)

C. *Hepatic and renal dysfunction*
D. *Drugs*

VII. Other Endocrine Causes

A. *Adrenal hyperplasia, tumors, or insufficiency*
B. *Hyperthyroidism or hypothyroidism*
C. *Diabetes mellitus*
D. *Steroidal contraceptives*

VIII. Ovary

A. *Biochemical defects and ovarian insensitivity*
B. *Destructive lesions*
C. *Estrogen-producing and androgen-producing tumors*
D. *Premature menopause (ovarian failure)*

IX. Uterus

A. *Endometrial destruction (Asherman's syndrome)*
B. *Cervical stenosis*

Developmental anomalies occasionally cause primary amenorrhea. In such cases, the diagnosis is usually obvious, as with an *imperforate hymen*. This lesion and *vaginal atresia* may result in uterine bleeding that cannot escape from the body (*cryptomenorrhea*).

Knowledge of normal development of the genitourinary system is prerequisite to understanding the numerous anatomic malformations that may cause amenorrhea or otherwise interfere with reproductive function. The urinary and reproductive systems develop from the intermediate mesoderm (p. 35). During folding, the intermediate mesoderm migrates ventrally and forms two longitudinal masses named the nephrogenic cords, which produce the urogenital ridges.

Three sets of excretory organs develop in human embryos. The first is the pronephros, which appears in human embryos

TABLE 12. Diagnosis of Amenorrhea

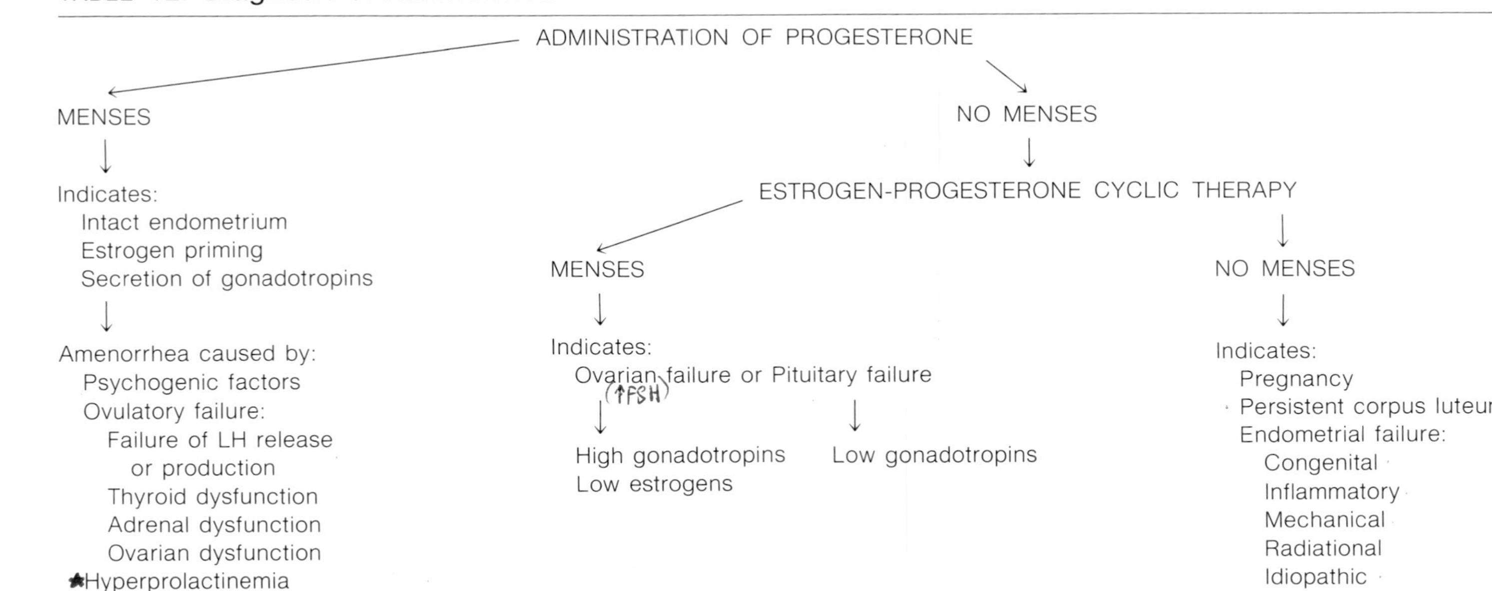

on day 22. Its regression is complete by the beginning of the fifth week. It consists of several pairs of tubules and a pronephric duct. Caudad to the pronephros, the blind end of the pronephric duct continues to grow toward the cloaca, which it perforates on about day 30. The mesonephros appears during the fourth week, caudad to the pronephros. Clusters of cells within the nephrogenic cord differentiate into S-shaped mesonephric tubules, which become continuous with the pronephric duct, which at this stage is designated the mesonephric duct. The medial end of each tubule expands, is invaginated by capillaries, and forms a glomerulus. By the tenth week most of these tubules have degenerated. A few caudal tubules persist as genital ducts in men or as vestigial structures in women. The metanephros, or adult kidney, develops from the ureteric bud and the metanephrogenic mass. The ureteric bud, which arises during the fifth week from the mesonephric duct just anterior to the cloaca, gives rise to the ureter, renal pelvis, calyces, and all the collecting ducts of the adult kidney. Mesenchymal cells from the metanephrogenic mass form a cap over the blind end of each newly formed collecting duct. Clusters of cells in each cap differentiate into Bowman's capsule and its associated tubules to form a nephron. Communication is then established between nephron and collecting duct. By early in the third month the fetal kidney has become functional. The mature fetus may void as much as 450 ml/day into the amniotic sac. During development the kidneys rise out of the pelvis to a site opposite the future second lumbar vertebra.

The cloaca, a common endodermal chamber, is divided into a dorsal rectum and a ventral region comprising bladder and urogenital sinus. The apex of the bladder tapers to form an elongate tube, the urachus, which is continuous at the umbilicus with the proximal remnant of the allantois. After birth the urachus persists as the median umbilical ligament.

Sex cannot be ascertained in the human embryo until approximately the sixth to seventh week. In early development the genital systems in both sexes are similar and potentially bisexual. This indifferent stage persists from the fifth to the seventh week of development.

The gonads are derived from three sources: celomic epithelium of the urogenital ridge, the underlying mesenchyme, and the primordial germ cells. A bulge on the medial side of the mesonephros forms the gonadal ridge. The celomic epithelium gives rise to primary sex cords, which grow into the underlying mesenchyme. The primordial germ cells are first seen early in the fourth week in the wall of the yolk sac near the origin of the allantois. They migrate along the dorsal mesentery of the hindgut into the gonadal ridge. During the sixth week they are incorporated into the primary sex cords.

In embryos with a Y chromosome, the seminiferous cords form branches the ends of which anastomose to form the rete testis. Mesonephric tubules that communicate with the mesonephric (wolffian) duct give rise to the efferent ductules, whereas the mesonephric duct forms the epididymis and ductus (vas) deferens. Mesenchymal elements give rise to the interstitial cells of Leydig.

In embryos that lack a Y chromosome, gonadal development occurs slowly. The primary sex cords do not become prominent but they form a rudimentary rete ovarii. During the fourth month the definitive cortex of the ovary first appears. The germinal epithelium produces the secondary sex cords, or cortical cords, which incorporate primordial germ cells.

The paramesonephric (müllerian) duct first appears during the sixth week as a groove in the thickened epithelium on the lateral aspect of the urogenital ridge. The groove never closes at its cephalic end but remains open to the celomic cavity. Distally the edges of the groove fuse to form the paramesonephric duct, which runs parallel to the mesonephric duct. Caudally the paramesonephric ducts cross ventrad to the mesonephric ducts, fusing in the midline into a Y-shaped uterovaginal primordium. This primordium reaches the urogenital sinus during the eighth week, producing an elevation named the müllerian tubercle.

In the presence of ovaries, the paramesonephric ducts develop into the female genital tract. The cranial longitudinal segments form the oviducts, their ostia becoming the fimbriated extremities. The uterus develops from the middle transverse portion of the paramesonephric duct as a result of proliferation of cells in this region and elevation of the cranial aspect of the uterovaginal primordium. The cervix and part of the vagina develop from the caudal longitudinal segment of the paramesonephric duct. The caudal tip of the uterovaginal primordium proliferates to produce a solid vaginal cord. Paired sinovaginal bulbs grow from the urogenital sinus and fuse with the vaginal cord. This solid cord of endodermal and mesodermal cells forms the vaginal plate. The central cells of this plate subsequently break down and form the lumen of the vagina, part or all of which is lined by endodermal cells derived from the sinovaginal bulbs.

In the female, buds grow out from the urethra into the surrounding mesenchyme to form the urethral and paraurethral (Skene's) glands. Similar outgrowths from the urogenital sinus form the greater vestibular (Bartholin's) glands.

The entire mesonephric system undergoes atrophy in the female. The cranial group of tubules persists as a functionless vestige, the epoophoron, which is located within the mesosalpinx. The caudal group of mesonephric tubules forms the small paroophoron, which usually disappears before adult life. Vestiges of the caudal portion of the mesonephric duct (Gartner's duct) may be found anywhere between the epoophoron and the hymen.

During the indifferent stage of genital development, the mesoderm surrounding the cloacal membrane undergoes proliferation (at about the fourth week), producing, cranially, the genital tubercle, and, laterally, the labioscrotal swellings and urogenital folds. The phallus develops as the genital tubercle elongates. The rectouterine septum fuses with the cloacal membrane at the end of the sixth week. Rupture of this membrane forms the anus and the urogenital opening.

The external female genitalia develop during the ninth to twelfth weeks. The phallus develops into the clitoris, with glans and prepuce. The urogenital folds, which form the labia minora, do not fuse except in front of the anus. Laterally, the labioscrotal folds, which form the labia majora, remain unfused except posteriorly, to form the posterior labial commissure, and anteriorly, to form the mons pubis.

Of the numerous malformations of the genital tract from the external genitalia to the uterus, only a few will prevent or conceal menstruation. In children, agglutination of the labia may be confused with an imperforate hymen. The simplest effective treatment is gentle digital separation of the adhesions and the local use of vaseline or estrogen creams.

A true imperforate hymen at the onset of menses will result in retention of blood within the vagina (hematocolpos), uterus (hematometra), and fallopian tube (hematosalpinx), and even the peritoneal cavity. Treatment is incision of the hymen and sometimes excision of a wedge of tissue. Ultimate fertility is preserved if the tubes are not damaged by the collections of blood.

Aplasia of the vagina may be associated with absence of the uterus and anomalies of the urinary tract. If the uterus is normal, fertility may be restored after reconstruction of a vaginal canal.

A transverse septum of the vagina may be mistaken for congenital absence of the vagina. A longitudinal septum has no effect on menses or fertility in general. Aplasia of the vagina results from agenesis of the vaginal cord. Atresia results from failure of canalization (p. 203).

Most anomalies of the uterus result from agenesis, aplasia, or abnormalities of differentiation, regression, or fusion of the müllerian ducts. In the case of aplasia, a cord of connective tissue replaces the uterus. This malformation is usually accompanied by vaginal anomalies. Only a few of the uterine malformations are clinically significant.

A unicornuate uterus, which results from aplasia of one müllerian duct, is not clinically important. A noncommunicating rudimentary horn may collect blood to form an enlarging mass. In a septate uterus, fusion is complete but the septum persists. In a bicornuate uterus, fusion occurs only in the lower portion of the müllerian ducts, resulting in a single cervix and a single vagina. With complete duplication of the müllerian ducts (uterus didelphys), the uterus and cervix are double and the vagina is septate. The ovaries are normal, however, and there is no disturbance of menstruation.

Chromosomal and genetic causes of amenorrhea include several fairly common disorders such as *gonadal dysgenesis* and *testicular feminization* and a great variety of *hermaphroditic and intersexual syndromes,* some of which reflect *specific biochemical defects.*

Gonadal dysgenesis frequently presents clinically as *Turner's syndrome*. The chromosomal pattern is usually XO or mosaic and the *sex chromatin* is usually *negative.* These patients have *high levels of gonadotropins* and *low levels of estrogen and lack secondary sexual characteristics.* Classically these girls are short, with low-set ears and a webbed neck. Typically there are "*streak gonads.*" The müllerian ducts form, but the uterus and tubes remain prepuberal. The external genitalia are female and the children are usually reared as girls.

Diagnosis is suspected on clinical grounds and confirmed by *karyotype,* analysis of X (Barr) and Y (fluorescent chromosome) *bodies,* and *laparoscopy.* Differential diagnosis includes ovarian hypoplasia, delayed puberty, and pituitary dwarfism. Treatment with *estrogens* should be *delayed* until around age 14 to prevent premature closure of the epiphyses.

Patients with Turner's syndrome often have in addition nevi, coarctation of the aorta, a shield chest, and edema at birth. FSH and LH levels are elevated and estrogen is decreased; 17-ketosteroids, 17-hydroxycorticoids, and ACTH are within normal limits.

Of all patients with an XO chromosomal constitution only about 25% are born alive. Certain patients with Turner's syndrome may have an iso-X or a ring chromosome and a positive sex chromatin (Barr body). In cases of gonadal dysgenesis, arrest occurs before or immediately after gonadal differentiation. With gonadal agenesis, the entire gonadal anlage is missing. These patients may therefore have an XX or an XY chromosomal pattern, but they will be amenorrheic and their gender role will be female.

Klinefelter's syndrome is the commonest sex chromosomal anomaly. These phenotypic males have a chromosomal pattern of 47,XXY, atrophic testes, and oligospermia or azoospermia. They frequently have gynecomastia and some degree of mental retardation.

The 47,XXX "superfemale" may be a phenotypically normal woman. There is an increased incidence of mental retardation but the patients are sometimes fertile.

Testicular feminization is a fairly common cause of amenorrhea in *phenotypic females* with an XY chromosomal constitution. This disorder may be considered a form of intersexuality or *pseudohermaphroditism* (p. 208). The patients have *scanty sexual hair* (pubic and axillary) but may have moderately *well-developed breasts*. Because müllerian development is lacking, the uterus is absent or rudimentary, and oviducts are missing. *Testes may be abdominal, inguinal, or vulvar.* The vagina commonly ends in a blind pouch.

The main cause is probably a defect in *androgen receptors* in the *end organs*, although there may also be a defect in synthesis of androgen. Treatment is directed toward *removing the testes* because of the increased incidence of *neoplasia* in these ectopic gonads. *Estrogen therapy* should be continued permanently. It may be necessary to *construct a functional vagina* when the patient indicates a desire to initiate coitus.

In testicular feminization, 17-ketosteroids are within the male range but estrogenic effects resemble those of the normal female. Gonadotropin levels are variable. One form of the syndrome results from a deficiency in 5-alpha-reductase with failure of conversion of testosterone to dihydrotestosterone. These patients should not be told that they are genetic males, for their psychologic orientation and sex of rearing are female. In incomplete forms of the syndrome the external genitalia are ambiguous.

True hermaphrodites have both ovarian and testicular tissue, either in the form of one *ovary* and one *testis* or as bilateral *mixed gonads* containing both tissues. The hermaphrodite may have associated *anomalies of the urinary tract*. The most common chromosomal pattern is 46,XX and the sex chromatin is usually positive, but the phenotype depends on the predominant tissue. The external genitalia are usually ambiguous. Although these patients may menstruate, they are usually infertile.

The *female pseudohermaphrodite* has *ovaries*, but the genital ducts and external genitalia differentiate to some extent along male lines. The *male pseudohermaphrodite* has *testes*, but the genital ducts, external genitalia, or both differentiate to some extent in the female direction.

Sexual differentiation depends on *genetic* and *environmental* factors. A discrepancy among the various criteria of sexual identification results in intersexuality.

Criteria of sexuality include chromosomal pattern, sex chromatin, gonadal structure, differentiation of the genital ducts (internal genitalia), external genitalia, hormonal status, sex of rearing, and gender role (psychologic orientation). Since the *sex of rearing* is crucial to the psychologic development of the child and is well established after the second year of life, it is important to *assign sex* definitively as *early* as possible. Normal morphologic development of the urogenital system is described on pages 199 through 203.

All fetuses are potentially bisexual. In the fourth week of gestation an indifferent gonad appears in both sexes. Gonadal differentiation occurs at about the sixth week. Normally a Y chromosome leads to the development of a testis, which in turn produces a male phenotype, with certain exceptions such as testicular feminization. The primordia differentiate into the internal genitalia, or genital ducts, at about the seventh week. Testes produce an androgenic steroid, which stimulates the wolffian ducts and induces the development of male external genitalia. The testes normally produce also a nonsteroid (Factor X, or müllerian inhibiting factor), which inhibits the müllerian ducts. In normal female differentiation the wolffian ducts regress and the müllerian ducts develop into uterus, oviducts, and possibly a portion of the upper vagina. Normal sexual development requires appropriate stimulation of one ductal system and repression of the other. Development of the external genitalia is hormonally determined.

Clinical investigation of the child with ambiguous genitalia should occur in a systematic sequence. A history of the pregnancy with special reference to *drugs or hormones* ingested by the mother should be obtained. *Physical examination* of the infant should record associated anomalies, as in Turner's syndrome (p. 205), or small testes, as in Klinefelter's syndrome (p. 205). Small testes in a virilized male infant may suggest the adrenogenital syndrome (p. 209). A *buccal smear* should be obtained for analysis of sex chromatin and a *karyotype* performed to detect aneuploidy and mosaicism. *Urethroscopy* or injection of contrast medium into the "vagina" or urogenital sinus should reveal the internal genitalia.

Hormonal studies may provide diagnostic information. For example, 17-ketosteroid levels are elevated in the congenital adrenogenital syndrome, whereas they are normal if the masculinization results from exogenous androgens transferred from the maternal circulation. In certain cases *laparotomy* with *biopsy* of the gonads may be required for definitive diagnosis. *Intravenous pyelography* should be performed to detect associated anomalies of the urinary tract.

Two primarily psychiatric problems should be distinguished from hermaphroditism. In the transsexual patient there are no discrepancies among the anatomic criteria of sex, but the patient feels "trapped in the body of the wrong sex." Such patients may request surgical change of gender. These extensive operations should be performed only after psychiatric evaluation.

A transvestite is a patient who derives pleasure from wearing the clothes of the opposite sex. These patients do not request operations to change their sex. When their behavior conflicts with the law, they require psychiatric care. Neither transvestites nor transsexuals are necessarily homosexual.

Female pseudohermaphroditism in the newborn may be caused by congenital *adrenal hyperplasia*, which produces an excess of adrenal *androgens* and the *congenital adrenogenital syndrome*. Other causes include *masculinizing tumors* of the mother's *ovary* and *exogenous hormones* administered to the mother during pregnancy. Since it is hazardous to change the gender role later in life, in cases of doubt these children should be *raised as girls*.

Virilization is less severe when the adrenogenital syndrome occurs after puberty. Identical phenotypic effects may be produced by *hyperplasia, adenoma*, and *carcinoma* of the *adrenal cortex*. The basic defect is a *deficiency in the enzymes* required for the synthesis of cortisol. Because of negative feedback, ACTH levels are elevated. The resulting excess adrenal androgen blocks production of FSH and LH and causes virilization (Table 13).

In the *adrenogenital syndrome*, the external genitalia are masculinized, but the uterus and fallopian tubes are normal. The chromosomal pattern is 46,XX and the *sex chromatin* is *positive*. Primary amenorrhea may occur on a hormonal basis. 17-Ketosteroids are elevated and precocious growth may occur until the age of 10 to 11, at which time the patients cease to grow. Ultimately they are shorter than normal because of premature closure of the epiphyses. The *treatment* is cortisone to suppress ACTH and, in turn, adrenal androgen. *Plastic surgical procedures* may be required if the external genitalia are significantly masculinized.

The adrenogenital syndrome stems from a defect in enzymatic hydroxylation in the zona fasciculata of the adrenal cortex. Negative feedback results in increase in ACTH, which in turn stimulates the zona reticularis to produce androgen. In the most common form of the syndrome a block in 21-hydroxylase results in an increase in pregnanetriol in the urine. Other enzymatic defects are less specifically associated with the adrenogenital syndrome.

A variety of *neoplastic, inflammatory,* and *destructive* lesions in the *brain, hypothalamus,* or *pituitary* may be associated with amenorrhea with or without other endocrine stigmata. A basophilic adenoma of the pituitary may produce *Cushing's syndrome,* although a lesion of the adrenal gland is the more common cause. Chromophobe adenomas also may produce amenorrhea.

Several eponyms are applied to the *amenorrhea-galactorrhea* syndromes. The *Chiari-Frommel syndrome* of persistent *postpartum* amenorrhea and galactorrhea is perhaps typical of the group. It probably represents *hypothalamic dysfunction*, for no organic lesion has been identified. Estrogens and gonadotropins are markedly depressed. Amenorrhea and galactorrhea persisting for six months or more postpartum, as well as the nonpuerperal varieties of this syndrome, should be referred for

TABLE 13. Diagnosis of Ovulatory Failure

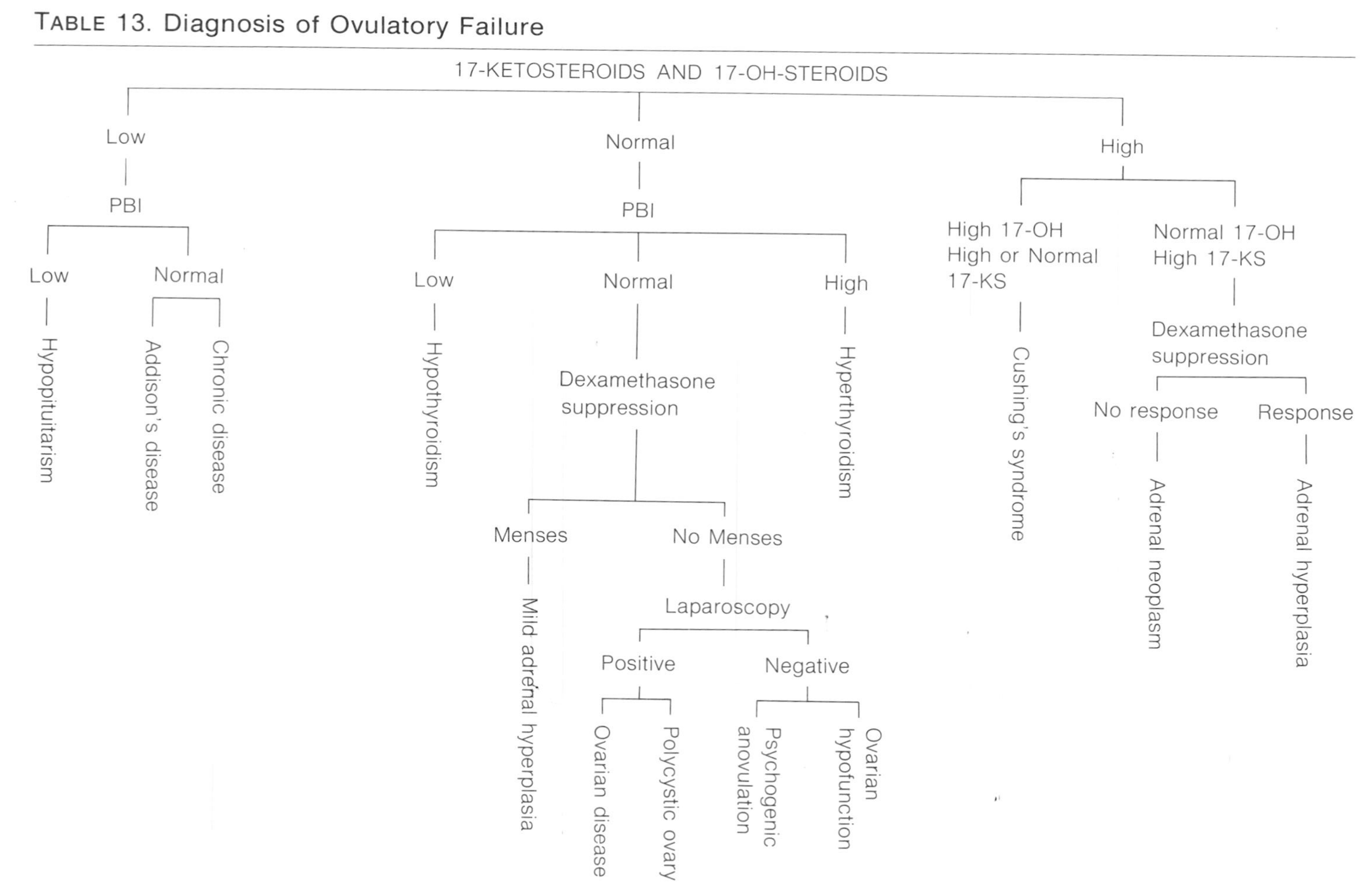

diagnosis and treatment. Amenorrhea-galactorrhea syndromes associated with *hyperprolactinemia* are often successfully treated with *bromocriptine mesylate*. *Pituitary adenomas* must be ruled out in patients with hyperprolactinemia. The hormonal control of lactogenesis and galactopoiesis are described on page 69.

Selective deficiencies in production of gonadotropins may lead to *hypogonadotropic hypogonadism* or eunuchoidism. This disorder provides the classic indication for *gonadotropin therapy*. Complications of the therapeutic use of these hormones for any cause include *ovarian cysts* and *plural gestations*. The differential diagnosis of hypogonadotropic hypogonadism includes tumors of the pituitary, Sheehan's syndrome, and psychogenic amenorrhea.

Pituitary insufficiency may result from *Sheehan's syndrome*. This form of panhypopituitarism is often related to *shock* in abortion, labor, delivery, or the puerperium. It may result from thrombotic lesions in the pituitary. The combinations of tropic deficiencies resemble those in *Simmond's disease*, which is not related to complications of pregnancy.

The *polycystic ovary (Stein-Leventhal) syndrome* characteristically includes *bilateral pearly white ovaries*. These patients have amenorrhea or oligomenorrhea with anovulatory irregular uterine bleeding and *infertility*. Some degree of hirsutism (p. 215) and moderate obesity are commonly associated. Diagnosis is made on the finding, by laparoscopy or laparotomy, of large white ovaries with numerous small cysts and a thickened capsule. Gonadotropins as well as 17-ketosteroids are frequently within normal range but are sometimes elevated. Inappropriate secretion of LH results in an elevated LH:FSH ratio. Dexamethasone does not suppress the androgens significantly in the Stein-Leventhal syndrome. The differential diagnosis includes mild adrenal hyperplasia and Cushing's syndrome. Success is sometimes achieved surgically by *wedge resection* of the ovary, but medical treatment by stimulation of ovulation with *clomiphene* is the method of choice.

Clomiphene (Clomid) is a nonsteroidal estrogen antagonist. It is indicated in the anovulatory patient who has follicular function and adequate endogenous estrogen but lacks cyclic stimulation by pituitary gonadotropins. The dosage must be carefully regulated to minimize the likelihood of cystic ovarian enlargement and multiple ovulations with resulting plural gestations. Chorionic gonadotropin may be added to induce ovulation in refractory cases. Its long half-life makes it more effective than LH for this purpose.

In patients with deficiencies in pituitary gonadotropins (serious hypothalamic-pituitary disease), human menopausal gonadotropin (hMG) is occasionally effective in inducing ovulation. This hormone, which is purified from the urine of postmenopausal women, consists mainly of FSH with a little LH. Overstimulation of the ovaries with hMG (Pergonal) is a serious drawback to the use of this hormone.

Polycystic ovarian disease is now considered to result from primary dysfunction of the hypothalamus and pituitary rather than the ovary. Overstimulation by gonadotropins is found in association with an excess of ovarian steroids, indicating that the sex hormones do not suppress the gonadotropins, as in normal feedback mechanisms. As a result, there is an exaggerated response to gonadotropins. Like Cushing's disease, the Stein-Leventhal syndrome represents increased pituitary activity in conjunction with a paradoxical excess of the target hormone. The rationale for use of clomiphene is the blockage of the action of estrogen at the level of the hypothalamus.

The elevated level of LH may result from an increased pituitary response to estradiol (increased positive feedback). There may be in addition an increased pituitary response to luteinizing hormone-releasing hormone. The histologic changes in the ovaries are related to increased levels of androgens.

Amenorrhea after discontinuing *oral contraceptives* is uncommon in proportion to the number of women using these drugs. It results from *oversuppression of the pituitary and hypothalamus* and usually resolves spontaneously. Ovulation and menses may occasionally be induced by clomiphene. In order to attribute amenorrhea to oversuppression, pregnancy and tumors of the brain and pituitary must be ruled out.

Psychogenic causes of amenorrhea include psychosis, severe emotional shock, pseudocyesis (false, or spurious, pregnancy), and anorexia nervosa. In *anorexia nervosa,* unlike Sheehan's syndrome, no organic lesion of the pituitary is found, and thyroid and adrenal functions are not depressed. The patient with anorexia nervosa is cachectic and hypotensive. The underlying emotional problem may respond to *psychotherapy.*

A variety of *chronic diseases* such as tuberculosis and *nutritional deficiencies* may cause oligomenorrhea or amenorrhea. *Hepatic or renal dysfunction* also may interfere sufficiently with the metabolism of hormones to prevent normal menstruation. Many *drugs* in addition to hormones may depress menstrual function. The commonest etiologic agents are *phenothiazines* and *narcotics.*

Dysfunction of the *other endocrine organs* may also interfere with menstrual function. Adrenal hyperplasia, neoplasms, or insufficiency (Addison's disease) may lead to amenorrhea.

Unlike congenital adrenal hyperplasia, Cushing's syndrome represents hyperfunction of the zona fasciculata as well as the zona reticularis. Cushing's syndrome classically includes obesity, amenorrhea, hirsutism, and hypertension. Corticosteroids are elevated, whereas 17-ketosteroids may be normal or slightly elevated. In this syndrome overreaction to ACTH occurs, and the adrenal cortex cannot be suppressed with cortisone. Loss of diurnal fluctuation in the level of cortisol is found.

Hyperthyroidism as well as hypothyroidism may affect menstrual function unpredictably. Diabetes mellitus, particularly if untreated, also will adversely affect menstrual function. Aside from pregnancy, perhaps the commonest endocrine cause of decreased menses is ingestion of oral contraceptives. The patient should always be asked whether she has used these agents before other endocrine causes of amenorrhea are considered.

The *ovary* itself may be the cause of amenorrhea as a result of *biochemical defects, insensitivity* to tropic hormones, or *destructive lesions.* Functioning tumors of the ovary also may produce menstrual abnormalities including amenorrhea. Androgen-producing tumors (arrhenoblastoma, hilus cell tumor, and adrenal rest tumor) and estrogen-producing varieties (granulosa cell and theca cell tumors) may all cause amenorrhea or other menstrual abnormalities.

Premature menopause is defined as cessation of ovarian

function before the age of 40. This *ovarian failure* may result from premature aging of the ovaries or may follow prolonged lactation, debilitating diseases, or serious infections. Finally, the uterus itself may be the cause of amenorrhea. Uterine trauma sufficient to destroy the endometrium may occur after infection or overvigorous curettage (*Asherman's syndrome*). The intrauterine synechiae may occasionally be treated successfully by gentle curettage.

Cervical stenosis, which may also result from trauma, prevents the escape of menstrual blood. It may be treated by cervical dilatation.

Diagnosis of the cause of amenorrhea can often be made by careful history and physical examination alone. If pregnancy, chronic disease, and drug-induced amenorrhea are ruled out, the patient should usually be referred to a gynecologic endocrinologist.

The simplest tests to perform in the diagnosis of secondary amenorrhea are *endometrial biopsy,* hormonal *cytologic smear* of the vagina, and *buccal smear* for sex chromatin. Additional procedures that should be performed early in the investigation include full *dilatation and curettage, hysterosalpingography, hormonal assays,* and *culdoscopy* or *laparoscopy.*

Since amenorrhea may stem from central, systemic, or local causes, the remainder of the diagnostic investigation depends on assigning the etiologic factor to one of these groups.

To rule out a lesion in the central nervous system, electroencephalography, roentgenography of the skull, and testing of visual fields should be performed. In addition, the FSH level should be measured. The administration of metyrapone (metopirone) may be used as a test of pituitary function. This drug by interfering with 11-hydroxylation creates a negative feedback that stimulates a normal pituitary gland, as indicated by an increase in 17-hydroxycorticosteroids.

Computerized axial tomography (CAT) is useful in investigations of pituitary dysfunction. Hyperprolactinemia is often the clue to pituitary tumors. Tests of pituitary function include the response to insulin-induced hypoglycemia (which normally results in increases in growth hormone and ACTH), to TRH (which normally results in increases in TSH and prolactin), and to LRH (which normally results in increases in LH and FSH).

Peripheral and systemic lesions are investigated by measurement of protein-bound iodine, basal metabolic rate, dexamethasone suppression test, glucose tolerance test, analysis of 17-ketosteroids and 17-hydroxysteroids, erythrocyte sedimentation rate, leucocyte count, and hematocrit. Certain local factors can be ruled out by means of uterine sounding, curettage, and hysterography.

The *treatment* of secondary amenorrhea is determined by the *etiologic factor* and the *reproductive desires* of the patient. Diagnosis and correction of the disorder rather than the induction of menstruation are the primary goals. It is not necessary to induce ovulation except in patients who want to become pregnant.

Defeminization, Virilization, and Hirsutism

Defeminization, the relative loss of female sexual characteristics, usually precedes *virilization,* or masculinization. Defeminization involves diminution in mammary tissue and female distribution of fat, amenorrhea, and ovarian failure. Virilization is the development of male secondary sexual characteristics in a woman as a result of stimulation of the responsive tissues by excessive androgen. A common sequence of masculinization is deepening of the voice, hirsutism, a male pattern of baldness, increased secretion of sebaceous glands with occasional acne, hypertrophy of the clitoris, and increased muscle mass.

Hirsutism is the excessive growth of hair on the body or face of a woman, usually involving the upper lip, chin, chest, abdomen, or legs. The major causes are listed in Table 14. Genetic, familial, and racial predispositions are the most common etiologic factors in hirsutism. Hairiness, or hypertrichosis, is more common in Mediterranean races, for example. It is therefore

TABLE 14. Etiology of Hirsutism

I. Genetic, Familial, or Racial

II. Pituitary-Hypothalamic

A. *Acromegaly*
B. *Cushing's syndrome*
C. *Polycystic ovary syndrome*

III. Other Endocrine Defects

A. *Adrenogenital syndrome (congenital or acquired)*
B. *Cushing's syndrome*
C. *Adenoma and carcinoma of the adrenal*
D. *Hypothyroidism in children*

IV. Ovarian

A. *Masculinizing tumors*
B. *Menopause*

V. Systemic Physical and Emotional Illnesses

A. *Porphyria*
B. *Anorexia nervosa*

VI. Local Effects

A. *Plaster casts*
B. *Roentgen therapy*

VII. Drug-Induced

A. *Dilantin*
B. *Androgens*
C. *Corticosteroids*
D. *Diazoxide*

necessary in such people to compare the patient with other members of her family. In this idiopathic form of hirsutism the 17-ketosteroids and plasma testosterone levels are within normal limits.

Hirsutism of some degree is noted in many syndromes involving amenorrhea of central, constitutional, or peripheral origin, such as the polycystic ovary, Cushing, and adrenogenital syndromes. Most of the causes of hirsutism are discussed elsewhere in this Unit under the appropriate syndromes. Hirsutism caused by adrenal hyperplasia can be distinguished from that resulting from adrenal neoplasms in that the elevated 17-ketosteroids in adrenal tumors are not suppressed by the administration of *dexamethasone* (p. 213). Elevated levels of dehydroisoandrosterone suggest an adrenal source of excess androgens.

Menopause

Menopause is the cessation of menstruation for a year or more. It is caused by *ovarian failure* and is frequently preceded by anovulatory bleeding. It occurs normally between the ages of 40 and 55 and is often accompanied by the symptoms of the *climacteric,* including hot flashes, excessive perspiration, and depression or agitation. Menopause is frequently followed by endocrine and metabolic changes. Secretion of estrogens by the ovary is markedly decreased, although *peripheral conversion* of *adrenal steroids* to *estrone* continues after the menopause. Production of gonadotropin, mostly FSH, or *human menopausal gonadotropin* (hMG), is high in the early postmenopausal years. Later, *atrophy* of the introitus and the vagina, with occasional *dyspareunia* and *pruritus,* occur. Involution of the breasts is common. Atrophy of the epithelia of the genitourinary tract may predispose to cystitis, and in some women osteoporosis and cardiovascular degeneration may occur.

It is probably unnecessary to treat the asymptomatic postmenopausal woman with estrogen and wiser to *treat* only women with *climacteric symptoms.* In evaluating and treating climacteric patients, *environmental stresses* associated with the postmenopausal era of life must be recognized, for not all the symptoms attributed to the menopause result from decline in ovarian function. Mild discomfort may be managed with *tranquilizers* and mild *sedation,* or these drugs may be used to *reduce* the dose of *estrogen.* Symptoms of *vasomotor instability* and *urogenital atrophy* with *pruritus* are indications for estrogen replacement.

Estrogen prevents accelerated loss of bone in young women after castration, but in postmenopausal women, aging is a more important determinant of loss of bone than is decreased secretion of estrogen. Low-dose estrogen treatment of postmenopausal women neither prevents nor increases the risk of arteriosclerotic cardiovascular disease or cerebrovascular accidents. It is not certain whether estrogen treatment in postmenopausal women causes an increased incidence of mammary tumors, but it is clear that such treatment does not prevent these tumors. Treatment with estrogen does, however, increase the risk of endometrial carcinoma in postmenopausal women (p. 177).

Estrogen may be used in doses sufficient to treat climacteric symptoms without stimulating the endometrium or causing postmenopausal bleeding. The estrogens should be used in the *smallest effective dose* and administered *cyclically* (20 to 25 days per month). Many gynecologists recommend the addition of a *progestational agent* for the last five days of the cycle of estrogen treatment. The treatment should be *tapered* and *discontinued* as soon as possible. All postmenopausal patients receiving estrogen should have frequent measurements of *blood pressure* to exclude the possibility of hormone-induced hypertension. Regular examinations of the *breast* are required. *Postmenopausal bleeding* demands the prompt exclusion of neoplastic diseases, particularly *carcinoma of the endometrium*.

Infertility

Infertility is diminished fertility, unlike *sterility*, which is absolute inability to reproduce. Female sterility is the inability to conceive. Male sterility is the inability to fertilize an ovum. *Primary infertility* means diminished fertility throughout the reproductive years, whereas *secondary infertility* implies one or more earlier successful pregnancies. Diagnosis of infertility is not made until failure to conceive has occurred despite 12 *months* or longer of *attempting pregnancy*. A female factor may be uncovered in not more than half the cases of infertility.

Male causes include impotence, failure to ejaculate, disturbances in numbers or motility of spermatozoa, and defective seminal plasma. *Female causes* include anovulation, tubal disease, or abnormalities of cervical mucus.

Anovulation is evaluated by means of a daily morning temperature graph (basal body temperature, or BBT), endometrial biopsy to demonstrate lack of a secretory endometrium, and inadequate cyclic changes in the cervical mucus or vaginal cytologic smear. The ovaries may be visualized directly by endoscopy.

Tubal disease (occlusion or lack of peristalsis) may be evaluated by three means. The simplest is insufflation of CO_2 through the cervix (Rubin's test, p. 131). This test is best performed on days 6 to 14 of the cycle. Patency of the tubes is suggested by shoulder pain (diaphragmatic irritation). The second technique, which provides much more information, is hysterosalpingography, in which contrast medium is injected into the cervix for visualization of the lumens of the uterus and tubes. The third technique is endoscopy (laparoscopy or culdoscopy), in which the tubes may be visualized directly while dye is injected through the cervix.

Abnormalities of cervical mucus are detected by careful examination of amount and quality throughout the cycle. The cervical mucus should exhibit a fern pattern in the first half of the cycle, and Spinnbarkeit (ability of the mucus to be drawn into long threads) should be maximal at ovulation. In a normal *Sims-Hühner (postcoital)* test, 10 or more motile spermatozoa per high-power field should be seen in cervical mucus at midcycle, two hours after coitus. In any investigation of infertility the *couple* should be *interviewed* together early and any *male factor ruled out* before complicated procedures are performed on the woman. *Ovulation, adequate production of sperm, patency of the fallopian tubes,* and a *histologically normal endometrium* may be detected by relatively simple means. Further diagnosis and treatment usually require *referral.*

Common male factors are defects in number, motility, or proportion of morphologically normal spermatozoa. In evaluation of the semen, the total ejaculate should be obtained, preferably by masturbation. In certain cases of oligospermia, a homologous insemination may be performed with the husband's semen. The use of a split ejaculate, in which only the first portion is used for insemination, is occasionally valuable in homologous insemination for oligospermia. The first portion, containing fluid from the prostate and Cowper's glands, contains most of the viable spermatozoa and can be effectively separated from the third portion, which contains fluid from the seminal vesicles. With azoospermia, a heterologous (donor) insemination may be the only alternative to adoption. Causes of male infertility include: congenital defects of the genitalia, such as cryptorchidism, testicular hypoplasia, absence of the vasa deferentia, hypospadias, and epispadias; acquired defects, such as varicocele, local infections and trauma, and neoplasms; physical and toxic factors, such as heat, radiation, and drugs; chromosomal aberrations, such as Klinefelter's syndrome with dysgenesis of the seminiferous tubules; retrograde ejaculation, of idiopathic or diabetic origin; neuropsychiatric problems; and nutritional and endocrine factors.

Semen for analysis should be collected after a period of abstinence of three to four days. The average volume after three days of abstinence is approximately 1 to 6 ml. Normally at least 60 to 80% of the sperm should be motile one hour after ejaculation. The normal sperm count varies between 40 and 125 million/ml. Counts under 20 million/ml reflect true oligospermia. In a fertile semen sample at least 60% of the cells are morphologically normal. The concentrations of fructose and citric acid in the semen are indices of function of the seminal vesicles and prostate, respectively. Complete absence of fructose in azoospermic men indicates congenital bilateral absence of the vasa deferentia, inasmuch as the seminal vesicles and the vas deferens arise from the same embryologic structures.

Ovulation may be detected by an estrogenic ("cornified") vaginal smear followed by a progestational smear. An increase in amount and a decrease in viscosity of cervical mucus at ovulation, followed by the disappearance of a fern, are correlated with a normal biphasic basal body temperature curve. The best evidence is provided by measurement of serum progesterone and an endometrial biopsy that shows secretory changes.

Ovulation may be detected in the laboratory by the preovulatory LH surge, the urinary estrogen peak 24 hours before ovulation, a total urinary gonadotropin peak just before ovulation, and pregnanediol excretion, which is a measure of production of progesterone by the corpus luteum.

Ovulatory defects may be detected and treated by induction of ovulation. Anovulation may result from a central nervous system, intermediate, or gonadal factor. The major causes are discussed in the section on amenorrhea (pp. 197–215).

Abnormal cervical mucus may create an environment "hostile" to the sperm. In the postcoital test, semen is aspirated from the vaginal pool and the endocervix shortly after intercourse to assess the motility of the spermatozoa.

Less commonly, infertility may stem from lesions of the vagina (anomalies or stenosis) or cervix (trauma, inflammation, stenosis, and incompetent os). Abnormalities of the corpus that occasionally lead to infertility include congenital anomalies, submucous myomas, and traumatic scarring of the endometrium (Asherman's syndrome), which may be treated by gentle curettage.

A luteal phase defect is often detectable by endometrial biopsy. In such cases either the endometrium is not responsive or the ovary produces insufficient progesterone. In this condition exogenous progesterone or hCG may be therapeutic. Inflammatory occlusions of the oviduct or adhesions may be treated surgically with moderate success, if the fimbriae and tubal peristalsis remain unimpaired. Tuberculosis must be ruled out during the investigation of female factors. Immunologic factors, such as antibodies to components of the semen, are difficult to treat.

Psychogenic factors are said to cause spasm of the reproductive tract on occasion. In rare instances, psychiatric treatment may be helpful.

Abnormal Uterine Bleeding

Abnormal or excessive uterine bleeding may result from *endocrine dysfunction,* but neoplasms and other *anatomic causes* and complications of pregnancy must be *ruled out* before hormonal therapy is initiated. *Dysfunctional uterine bleeding* (bleeding without an obvious anatomic abnormality) is usually *anovulatory.* It is most common shortly after the *menarche* or just before the *menopause,* but it may occur at other times as well.

Prolonged dysfunctional bleeding may result from a persistent graafian follicle. In such cases, withdrawal of estrogen leads to *delayed endometrial shedding* and irregular bleeding. The bleeding is caused by estrogenic overstimulation followed by withdrawal or diminution of estrogen, unopposed by progesterone. *Estrogenic stimulation* results in bleeding from a *proliferative or hyperplastic endometrium,* or occasionally from endometrial polyps or carcinoma. A related cause is "breakthrough bleeding" during the use of oral contraceptives.

Dysfunctional bleeding may result from disorders of the *central nervous system, pituitary,* or *ovary,* or from the effects of exogenous or endogenous *steroids.* Etiologic factors related to *systemic metabolic disorders* include hyperthyroidism, hypothyroidism, *hepatic dysfunction,* and a variety of *chronic diseases.* Bleeding from a *secretory endometrium,* which indicates *ovulation,* usually implies an *anatomic lesion* rather than an endocrine disorder. The investigation of ovulatory bleeding should include a *hysterogram* and *hematologic* studies. Anovulatory bleeding requires consideration of nutritional, metabolic, and emotional factors. Polycystic ovaries may be ruled out by culdoscopy or laparoscopy.

Most important, any abnormal bleeding in an adult requires *Papanicolaou smear and curettage before treatment.* For greatest accuracy of diagnosis, curettage is best performed just before menses. In an adolescent patient presumptive dysfunctional bleeding may be treated without curettage.

Ovulatory bleeding may occasionally produce minimal midcyclic bleeding in the absence of an organic lesion. Abnormal uterine bleeding may result from organic lesions of the ovary, oviduct, corpus, cervix, and vagina. Complications of pregnancy include ectopic gestation, abortion, bleeding corpus luteum, hydatidiform mole, and choriocarcinoma.

Genital causes unassociated with pregnancy include myomas, and carcinoma, polyps, or hyperplasia of the endometrium; chronic cervicitis; polyps and carcinomas of the cervix; carcinoma of the vagina; functional ovarian cysts; and functioning ovarian neoplasms.

Extragenital causes include blood dyscrasias, thrombocytopenia, deficient clotting factors, endocrinopathies, and, uncommonly, hypertension. In addition bleeding from the urinary tract and rectum must be excluded.

Treatment of uterine bleeding depends on the cause. In *adolescents, cyclic estrogen and progesterone therapy* may be instituted after a Papanicolaou smear without a preliminary curettage. If bleeding persists after cyclic estrogen-progesterone therapy (medical curettage), a complete diagnostic investigation including formal curettage is required. In cases of recurrent apparently dysfunctional bleeding in younger patients, progesterone may be used while the investigation continues.

Attempts to *induce ovulation* are justified only when *fertility* is part of the goal of therapy. In older patients who have completed their families, recurrent irregular bleeding may be treated by hysterectomy.

Dysmenorrhea

Dysmenorrhea, or painful menstruation, is a symptom and not a disease. Dysmenorrhea may be the commonest gynecologic symptom. It is the direct cause of the loss of countless woman-hours of work.

Primary dysmenorrhea occurs in the absence of a significant pelvic lesion. It is *essential*, or *functional*, dysmenorrhea and is caused by factors intrinsic to the uterus. Primary dysmenorrhea is the more common form of the symptom. Its onset is usually in *adolescence*, within two years of the menarche. The cause is unknown, but it is generally associated with *ovulatory cycles*. The patients are often tense, nonathletic, neurotic girls who are mother-dominated and have a low pain threshold. They are often poorly prepared for menarche and femininity. The *psychogenic component* is usually obvious. In the *secondary form*, *pelvic disease* can be demonstrated.

Common causes of secondary dysmenorrhea are *endometriosis, adenomyosis*, and *chronic pelvic inflammatory disease*. Even if palpable findings are absent on pelvic examination, endometriosis may still be the cause of the dysmenorrhea. It should therefore be ruled out by endoscopy. The secondary form begins in adult life, affecting a previously symptom-free woman.

The *treatment* of primary dysmenorrhea is necessarily *symptomatic*. It includes encouraging exercise and increasing extrafamilial interests and activities. Strong *reassurance* may be supplemented by mild *analgesics, psychic stimulants,* and *anticholinergic drugs,* but narcotics and strong analgesics should be avoided. Inasmuch as primary dysmenorrhea may be related to production of *prostaglandin,* therapy with *inhibitors* of prostaglandin is occasionally effective. *Retroprogestins* may relieve dysmenorrhea without necessarily inhibiting ovulation. In more severe cases, *ovulation may be inhibited* by oral contraceptive drugs or intramuscular injections of progestins. *Psychiatric evaluation* should be requested before drastic therapeutic procedures are undertaken. Presacral neurectomy is occasionally performed as a last resort for refractory cases.

Premenstrual Tension Syndrome

The *premenstrual tension syndrome* is a symptom complex occurring in the days or week before menstruation. It comprises tension, irritability, or depression, sometimes associated with tenderness or fullness of the breasts, abdominal bloating, headache, and edema. Etiologic factors include an *unstable personality, environmental stress,* and *cyclic changes in ovarian function.* The onset of the syndrome is usually in the fourth decade of life.

Premenstrual tension is associated with *ovulatory cycles.* In its severe form it may cause psychic and physical incapacitation of the woman for one third of the month. It is temporally related to an increase in crimes committed by women, accidents, and suicides. It may be associated with *secondary hyperaldosteronism,* causing retention of sodium and water and resulting edema and headache. Treatment includes strong *reassurance, antidepressant drugs,* and *diuretics,* particularly spironolactone. Severe emotional disturbances require referral to a *psychiatrist.*

UNIT VII

Control of Reproduction

Contraception

The *exponential increase* in the *populations* of the nation and the world has placed family planning and population control in the forefront of medical and social problems. The justification for detailed discussion of this subject is thus obvious.

Contraception may be either *temporary* or *permanent*. Permanent contraception is often referred to as *sterilization*. The *effectiveness* of a contraceptive technique is determined by the *pregnancy rate* (P. R.), which is defined as follows:

$$\text{P. R.} = \frac{\text{Number of pregnancies} \times 1{,}200}{\text{Patients observed} \times \text{months of exposure}}.$$

The pregnancy rate in a population that does not use contraception is about 80. The *birth rate* is the number of births per 1000 population. The *fertility rate* is the number of live births per 1000 female population between the ages of 15 and 44 years. The *marriage rate* is the number of marriages per 1000 population.

The estimated population of the world in mid-1975 was approximately four billion. With the 1975 birth rate of 26.6 and the death rate of 11.2, a rate of natural increase of 1.54% is achieved. That rate is equivalent to an increase of approximately 62 million people that year. For lesser developed regions, the rate of increase is about 2%, whereas for better developed countries such as the United States the rate is about 0.6%.

The effectiveness of a contraceptive is defined by its *theoretical effectiveness* and its *use-effectiveness*. Theoretical effectiveness is the antifertility action of any contraceptive method under *ideal conditions* with no omissions or errors in use. Use-effectiveness, or actual effectiveness, is the protection achieved under *realistic conditions* of life. It depends on motivation, cultural characteristics, and socioeconomic status of the population.

No ideal contraceptive is currently available. The characteristics of a perfect contraceptive include effectiveness, safety, low cost, esthetic qualities, ease of use, lack of relation to coitus, and absence of the requirement for repeated motivation.

Because patients are often receptive to discussions of contraception during pregnancy, it is wise to initiate these *discussions* during *pregnancy*, immediately post partum, and again at the six-week postpartum examination.

Contraception may be divided into *folk* (primitive), *conventional, modern,* and *experimental* methods. The important primitive techniques include coitus interruptus (withdrawal), extravaginal intercourse (including homosexual practices), abstinence, prolonged lactation, and postcoital douches.

Coitus interruptus, or *withdrawal,* is still a common practice throughout the world. Its pregnancy rate is 15. The contraceptive effectiveness depends on prevention of ejaculation into the vagina. It requires, however, male control over ejaculation and the prevention of the preejaculatory dribble of spermatozoa-laden discharge. The technique is often unsatisfying to one or both partners.

The *postcoital douche* as a sole means of contraception is to be discouraged because it has a failure rate almost equal to that of unprotected intercourse. The lack of effectiveness results from the very rapid entrance of the sperm into the cervical canal.

The failure rate of *prolonged lactation* as a contraceptive technique is unknown. The delay of ovulation post partum is highly variable and has been known to occur early during breastfeeding. The advantages of this technique are its lack of cost and ready availability.

Extravaginal intercourse is widely practiced, sometimes for purposes of contraception. Intertriginous, oral, and anal intercourse are effective only when not accompanied by vaginal intromission.

Abstinence is time-honored and effective but obviously inapplicable to most couples.

The *traditional* contraceptive techniques include rhythm; intravaginal chemicals such as jellies, creams, and foams; and mechanical methods including the condom, diaphragm, and cervical cap.

Aside from abstinence, the *rhythm* method is the only means of contraception in compliance with all religious doctrines. It depends on the avoidance of coitus at or near the time of ovulation, as indicated by a *rise in temperature* of about 0.7° F during the luteal phase of the cycle. Methods of detecting ovulation that are based on measurements of the viscosity of cervical mucus (p. 220) and its content of glucose are currently available. The pregnancy rate with this method is about 15. Because of uncertainties in the duration of viability of the sperm and the egg, intercourse must be avoided for a week before and three days after ovulation. The *success* of the method depends upon the *regularity of the menses* and requires *strong motivation.* For maximal safety, long periods of abstinence are required. Although menstruation occurs quite regularly at 14 days after ovulation, the length of the preovulatory phase is quite variable. Detection of the time of ovulation is therefore retrospective.

The use of *spermicidal jellies, creams,* and *foams* as the sole contraceptive technique is accompanied by a high pregnancy rate, which may approach 20. These agents may be used to advantage in the woman who has infrequent intercourse, but are unesthetic, must be used just before coitus, and may taste objectionable to those who perform cunnilingus. Allergic reactions to certain components of the products may occur in one or both partners. Preparations containing mercury may be teratogenic when used inadvertently in early pregnancy. Spermicidal agents are used most effectively in conjunction with the diaphragm. They are widely available without prescription.

A new preparation, the *Encare Oval,* provides a foaming, viscous barrier and contains a spermicide, nonoxynol-9. Pregnancy rates lower than those associated with traditional intravaginal spermicides have been reported from Europe but the data have not been confirmed in the United States. This product also is available without prescription.

The *vaginal diaphragm* is an occlusive device ordinarily varying from 65 to 90 mm in diameter. The pregnancy rate with the diaphragm alone is about 7, but it can be reduced by use in conjunction with a *spermicidal agent.* This form of contraception is inexpensive and it may render intercourse during menstrual periods more esthetic. The disadvantages of the diaphragm are the need for recurrent motivation, the association with coitus, and the requirement for fitting by a physician. For maximal effectiveness it is necessary to refit the diaphragm annually and post partum. Many women find the required vaginal manipulation unesthetic, but the sexual partner may be taught to insert the diaphragm. It may be inserted many hours before intercourse, but for maximal safety it should remain in place at least 8 hours after the last intercourse. This technique is not suitable with severe degrees of pelvic relaxation.

An occlusive technique that may be used in cases of vaginal relaxation is the cervical cap, which adheres by suction. The pregnancy rate with the cervical cap is about 7. Its principal disadvantage is the need for monthly removal but it requires no manipulations during the cycle.

Vaginal rings containing steroids and other preparations are in various stages of development, as is a collagen sponge that traps spermatozoa.

The *condom*, with a pregnancy rate of about 7, is still the most important traditional method of contraception throughout the world. It is also a mechanical device with an additional advantage of providing protection against venereal disease. Its principal disadvantages are the relatively high cost, the need for interruption of the sexual act, and the requirement for high motivation. Failures with the condom are related to poor timing of its application, breaks or leaks, and spillage of semen during removal. Some condoms decrease penile sensitivity, an effect that is generally considered a disadvantage.

The *intrauterine devices* (*IUDs*) regained popularity as contraceptives during the 1960s and early 1970s. The newer varieties are made of *inert plastics* or *stainless steel*. The pregnancy rate is about 2. The theoretical effectiveness is about 99% and the use-effectiveness about 97%. The mechanism of action is incompletely known, although the most popular current hypothesis involves an *antizygotic* or *antinidational* effect produced by a subclinical endometritis. Advantages include the low cost and the lack of relation to coitus. For further safety the patient should feel for the string, which projects through the cervix into the vagina. Additional protection is provided by use of a spermicidal agent at midcycle.

The disadvantages include difficulty of insertion of a standard-sized device in the nullipara and the possibility of uterine *perforation, bleeding,* and *cramps*, especially in the first few cycles. In addition there is a rate of initial *expulsion* of at least

10%. It is a *reversible* technique that involves only a *single decision* on the patient's part. It requires a physician or a physician's assistant to perform a pelvic examination to ascertain size and position of the uterus. The insertion is facilitated by application of a tenaculum to the anterior lip of the cervix. The larger devices have a lower rate of expulsion but generally cause more bleeding and cramps. The likelihood of uterine perforation is about 1 in 2000. *Open* (loop or coil) rather than closed (bow or ring) devices are used because perforation by the closed types is more likely to cause intestinal obstruction. An advance in the field of intrauterine contraception involved the addition of metallic *copper* to the plastic device. The ionization of the copper produces a spermicidal or antizygotic effect, which is in proportion to the amount of metal wrapped around the device. The FDA has recently ruled that these devices need be replaced only after three years.

Another intrauterine contraceptive technique involves the impregnation of the device with a slowly released steroid. The Progestasert device releases *progesterone* and combines the action of an inert IUD with local effects of the steroid on the endometrium. It too requires periodic removal and replacement by a new device. It has the further disadvantage of a possibly increased rate of ectopic pregnancy. Whether it will continue to be marketed is uncertain and its superiority over other IUDs remains questionable.

Since November, 1977, all IUDs, not just those containing metals or steroids, require *detailed* package *labeling* and a brochure, as are provided for oral contraceptives. *Contraindications* to the use of any IUD include pregnancy or suspicion of pregnancy; abnormalities of the uterus that cause distortion of the uterine cavity; acute pelvic inflammatory disease or a history of repeated bouts of pelvic inflammatory disease; postpartum endometritis or infected abortion in the preceding three months; known or suspected uterine or cervical cancer and abnormal Papanicolaou smears without histologic confirmation; genital bleeding of unknown cause; and untreated acute cervicitis. In addition, copper-containing devices are contraindicated in patients with Wilson's disease or a known allergy to copper.

Insertion of an IUD should be performed, if possible, during or shortly after a *menstrual period* to avoid placement within a pregnant uterus. To reduce the risk of perforation or expulsion, insertion after delivery or abortion should be delayed until the uterus has returned to its normal size. The patient with an IUD in place should receive an annual pelvic examination and Papanicolaou smear, although it is not necessary to remove the inert device periodically. For maximal protection it may be desirable to use another form of contraception for the first few months that the device is in place.

It was shown in 1976 that the IUD, contrary to earlier reports, *increases* not just the relative frequency of *ectopic pregnancy* with respect to all pregnancies, but the *absolute number* as well. This effect, which increases with duration of use of the IUD, is probably related to the *infection,* subclinical or overt, that the device produces. Unilateral nongonococcal *adnexal abscesses,* some of actinomycotic origin, have been described. Because of the risks of infection and ectopic pregnancy, it may be *inadvisable* to prescribe the IUD for a *nulligravida* to whom other contraceptive techniques are acceptable, or for a patient who has already had one ectopic pregnancy.

When a woman becomes pregnant with an IUD in place and wishes to keep the pregnancy, the device should be removed if the strings are visible. If the strings are not visible and the device cannot be removed readily, the patient is asked whether she wishes to continue with the pregnancy. If she does, she is informed of the increased risks of spontaneous abortion, infection, and ectopic pregnancy. If she does not want to continue with the pregnancy, the IUD is removed and the pregnancy is terminated. Intrauterine infection demands termination of the pregnancy in any case.

If a closed device or a copper-containing IUD perforates the uterus, it should be removed, by laparotomy or laparoscopy. An inert open device, however, is generally innocuous. The patient must be informed of its intraperitoneal location. If she does not request the removal of the inert device, it may remain in place as long as the patient is asymptomatic.

Hormonal contraception is the most effective form of birth control presently available. For the most part these drugs are used orally (*oral contraceptives*) but are also effective parenterally. Before any of these drugs is used a complete history and physical examination must be performed and pregnancy excluded. Particular attention must be paid to the breasts, the thyroid, and the blood pressure. A Papanicolaou smear should be obtained and the urine tested for protein and sugar. Young women should be examined at least annually and older women at even more frequent intervals.

The oral contraceptives are classified as either *combined* or *sequential* pills. The combined pills contain a synthetic *estrogen* and a *progestin*. The estrogen is either ethinyl estradiol or mestranol. Many preparations contain 35 μg of ethinyl estradiol or 50 μg of mestranol. Pills with larger doses of estrogen are also on the market. A variety of progestins is available, the most commonly used of which are norethynodrel and norethindrone, both nortestosterones. One group of progestins is related to androgens (C-19 nortestosterone); a second group is related to progesterone; and the third group has some intrinsic estrogenic activity.

The *effects* of the specific combined preparations depend on the *doses* and *ratios* of the estrogen and the progestin. All conventional combined oral contraceptives *inhibit ovulation*. They may also effect a change in *cervical mucus*, which results in decreased penetrability by spermatozoa. Furthermore, these drugs, particularly the combined preparations, may affect the *endometrium* or *tubal* and *uterine fluids*. In the combined form of oral contraception a pill containing estrogen and progestin is taken every day for *20 or 21* days starting on Day 5 of the cycle. Bleeding normally occurs three or four days after the last pill is taken. In the *21-day regimen* no pill is taken for 7 days. In the *28-day regimen* a placebo is taken for 7 days after the last active pill.

The sequential pills were withdrawn from use in the United States in 1976. In the sequential regimen estrogen alone is given in the first half of the cycle, and estrogen and progestin together in the second half. The alleged advantage of this regimen is the closer simulation of normal ovarian and menstrual functions, but sequential pills are not so effective as the combined types. The higher content of estrogen, furthermore, may lead to a higher incidence of thromboembolism, and use of the sequential preparations has been associated with hyperplastic and malignant lesions of the endometrium.

The advantages of all forms of oral contraception are their lack of relation to coitus and extreme effectiveness. The disadvantages are their relatively *high cost*, the need for *constant motivation*, the mild common *side effects*, and the rare but serious hazard of *thromboembolism* and other *cardiovascular complications*.

Mild and inconstant complications of the pill include nausea and occasional vomiting, bloating, enlargement and tenderness of the breasts, chloasma (irregular brownish discoloration of the skin of the face), weight gain, hypomenorrhea, benign cervical hyperplasia, post-pill amenorrhea (oversuppression syndrome), and altered metabolic functions, which may include increase in binding globulins, increase in Bromsulphalein retention, increase in triglycerides and total phospholipids, decrease in glucose tolerance, and possibly jaundice. There is an increase in coronary occlusion, a disease that is ordinarily rare in women of reproductive age.

Additional possible complications include a reversible hypertension (perhaps of the renin-dependent variety), uncommon neurologic or ophthalmologic problems, a change in libido (increase or decrease), and occasional increase in vaginal discharge.

Less common complications include an increase in gallbladder disease and urinary tract infections, presumably as a result of hormonal effects similar to those of pregnancy. Unusual complications, associated particularly with mestranol-containing compounds, are focal nodular hyperplasia of the liver and hepatic adenomas. Although most of the hepatic adenomas related to the pill are benign, they may rupture and produce serious hemorrhage.

The most serious complication that has been documented is thromboembolism, which may result from increased activity of *clotting factors* or perhaps a direct *vascular effect*.

The FDA requires greatly detailed information in the package labeling of oral contraceptives. All mortality and morbidity rates, however, must be compared with those associated with pregnancy itself. Furthermore, the seriousness of the cardiovascular complications is proportional to the prevalence of those diseases in the geographic area under consideration. The risks are therefore greater in western Europe and the United States than they are in most of Africa, for example, where the rate of thromboembolism is low.

Recent (1977) anterospective British studies report that the cardiovascular effects of oral contraceptives are synergistic, rather than simply additive, with those of hyperlipidemia, diabetes mellitus, hypertension, obesity, and cigarette smoking. The data from these studies, furthermore, indicate that the increased risk of death from cardiovascular disease in women is greater than that suggested in prior retrospective studies and it occurs at an age somewhat lower than previously reported. Women who have taken the pill for more than five years and who smoke are at particular risk. Again, diabetes, hypertension, and obesity add to the danger. These studies show that even if the pill is stopped, there is an increased likelihood of later death from cardiovascular disease. For women under the age of 35 there occurs only one death per year per 20,000 women on the pill. The risk rises sharply over this age. Between the ages of 35 and 44, the rate is one per 3000 women, and for women over the age of 45 the rate is one in 700. The overall annual rate is one death per 5000 women on the pill.

In addition to pulmonary embolism, myocardial infarction, and stroke, several other cardiovascular complications have been associated with the pill: subarachnoid hemorrhage, malignant hypertension, cardiomyopathy, mesenteric arterial thrombosis, and exacerbation of congenital and rheumatic cardiac diseases. Logical recommendations based on this new information are as follows. For women under the age of 30 there is no need to stop oral contraception, although cessation of smoking is advantageous. Between the ages of 30 and 35 the risk gradually increases. Some women in this group, for example those who have used oral contraceptives continuously for five years and smoke cigarettes, should reconsider the use of the pill. Nonsmokers could probably continue the pill. Women over the age of 35, particularly those who have used the pill continuously for five years or more or who smoke, would do well to consider other forms of contraception. Inasmuch as the pill takes several years to affect the cardiovascular system, there is no reason to stop it suddenly. The pill should not be stopped without an alternative temporary contraceptive method or sterilization.

Except for a history of a *thromboembolic disorder* or actual *thrombophlebitis, contraindications* to the pill are *relative.* There are no data to support the relation of combined oral contraceptives to the development of carcinoma of the corpus or cervix, although a carcinogenic effect may require a full generation to manifest itself. A recent (1977) prospective study, however, of women with dysplasia of the cervix showed an increase in severity of dysplasia and of conversion to carcinoma in situ in users of the contraceptive pill compared with users of other nonbarrier contraceptive methods. These data require confirmation.

The oral contraceptives must not be used in a patient with undiagnosed uterine bleeding and should be prescribed with increasing caution in older patients.

Among the contraindications are cardiovascular and venous diseases including varicose veins, hepatic disorders, a strong familial history of thromboembolism, diabetes, migraine headaches, hypertension, and myomas. The pill should not be used during lactation because steroids excreted in the milk may cause jaundice in the newborn.

The main cause of *failure* of oral contraception is *irregular or incorrect use* of the pills. With this form of birth control the use-effectiveness is considerably lower than the theoretical effectiveness. The pregnancy rate based on theoretical effectiveness of the combined pills is 0.1, or almost 100% effective. The pregnancy rate based on use-effectiveness, however, is 0.7.

The patient should not depend on the oral contraceptives for complete protection for the first 7 to 10 days of their use, but should use additional spermicidal agents or mechanical devices. If one pill is missed or if breakthrough bleeding occurs, the dosage should be doubled. If two pills are missed in sequence, some other form of contraception should be used for the remainder of that cycle. If no bleeding occurs by seven days after the last pill, a new cycle of medication should be started as though bleeding had occurred. If two or more amenorrheic cycles occur in succession, the pill should be stopped and the possibility of pregnancy investigated.

The pill should be taken from the fifth to the twenty-eighth day of the cycle and begun again on the fifth day after the onset of bleeding, or on the fifth day of amenorrhea if no bleeding has occurred during that cycle. It is advisable to take the pill at the same time each day. If one pill is forgotten, it should be taken as soon as possible after the regular time and the next pill at the regular time. If two pills in succession are forgotten, two pills should be taken as soon as possible after remembering and two pills at the regular time on the next day. Another form of contraception should be used for the remainder of that cycle. If three pills in succession are missed, a different procedure is advised. No additional pills should be taken. The patient is advised to wait four days longer and resume the medication regardless of whether the absence of hormones for seven days has resulted in uterine bleeding and even if the bleeding is still in progress. During the seven days that no pills have been taken and during the first ten days of the new cycle an additional form of contraception is required for maximal safety.

Slight spotting during the cycle, especially during the first two months of use, is not necessarily a contraindication to the pill. A tampon may be worn during the time of uterine spotting and a different pill prescribed. If the bleeding is equal in amount to a normal period, the pill should be stopped and a cycle of 21 pills begun on the fifth day, counting Day 1 as the first day of bleeding. If such heavy bleeding occurs twice, the patient should consult her physician. If a period is missed after proper use of 21 pills, it is most unlikely that pregnancy has occurred and the next cycle should be resumed on the eighth day after taking the last pill of the preceding cycle. If two periods in succession are missed, an examination is indicated to rule out pregnancy and possibly to switch medication.

Most of the side effects of the pill are mild, reversible, and related to the dosages of the steroids. The following less common but more serious complications require medical advice: cramps or swelling of the legs, chest pain, hemoptysis, dyspnea, sudden severe headache, dizziness, difficulty with vision or speech, and weakness or numbness of the extremities.

Many drugs in common use interfere with the action of oral contraceptives. The more important of these drugs include ampicillin, penicillin V, neomycin, phenobarbital, rifampicin, phenytoin, and phenylbutazone.

After a prolonged withholding of its approval, the Food and

Drug Administration in December, 1972, approved the "minipill" for contraceptive use. This pill contains only a progestin (0.35 mg of norethindrone). Unlike other oral contraceptives it is administered continuously in a daily dosage throughout the year. Its effectiveness is lower than that of either the conventional combined or sequential pills. The pregnancy rate is approximately 3 per 100 woman-years, compared with less than 1 for estrogen-progestin combinations.

Patients who have switched from conventional oral contraceptives to minipills have a lower rate of pregnancy than do those who have never been on oral contraceptives before taking the progestin-only medication. The rate of dropout for minipills is higher than that for conventional oral contraceptives, presumably because of a significant incidence of unpredictable bleeding that may not follow any consistent pattern even after prolonged use. The likelihood of thromboembolic complications associated with the minipill has not been ascertained although even this pure synthetic progestin has intrinsic estrogenic activity, which may increase the theoretical risk of thromboembolism.

The mode of action of the minipill is not clear, although it is known that it does not inhibit ovulation. For that reason the risk of ectopic pregnancy is increased. It may prevent the thinning at midcycle of the cervical mucus, preventing penetration by sperm, possibly affecting capacitation of sperm, or rendering the endometrium unfavorable for implantation. The advantages of the minipill have not yet been clearly demonstrated. They may possibly be associated with lower incidences of mild and serious complications of steroid contraception in general and they may be of value in very young girls in whom there is reluctance to suppress ovulation.

In 1973, estrogen-progestin preparations with 20 to 30 μg of estrogen were introduced. Their effectiveness is less than that of the conventional combined preparations but greater than that of the progestin-only pill.

Intramuscular contraception with long-acting progestins has been tested widely, but the Food and Drug Administration has withheld its approval of medroxyprogesterone acetate for routine contraception, mainly because of the finding of mammary tumors in beagles that had received large doses of chlormadinone, a related drug. Medroxyprogesterone acetate, however, in doses of 50 to 100 mg I.M. has been used widely for treatment of endometriosis (p. 159). The drug, given as a monthly injection or possibly even as an injection every three months in doses of 150 mg, could provide contraception for mental defectives and other women who cannot be relied upon to take a pill daily. It could also provide a logical alternative to sterilization for those women.

The differing proportions and dosages of the steroids in the conventional contraceptive formulations cause a variety of side effects. Fortunately, the drugs may be switched with ease, maintaining contraceptive effectiveness and minimizing the complications.

Signs of excess estrogen include nausea, edema, leg cramps, vertigo, leukorrhea, growth of myomas, chloasma, and uterine cramps. Estrogenic deficiency is manifested by irritability, nervousness, flushes, hot flashes, early and midcyclic bleeding, and decreased uterine bleeding.

Excess of progestins may be manifested by increased appetite and weight gain, fatigue, depression, acne, change in libido, jaundice, and hypomenorrhea. A deficiency of progestins may result in late breakthrough bleeding, heavy flow and clots, and delayed onset of the menses. The wide variety of combinations and dosages of estrogens and progestins usually permits the choice of a pill with minimal side effects and maximal effectiveness.

The "morning-after" pill is basically a high dose of an estrogen that can be used preferably within 24 hours and not later than 72 hours after unprotected intercourse. It is currently recommended in situations such as rape or other emergencies. The high dose of estrogen is often accompanied by nausea and vomiting. In February, 1973, the FDA approved the use of diethylstilbestrol in doses of 25 mg b.i.d. for five days as a morning-after pill. This is the most convenient estrogen to use as a postcoital contraceptive ("interceptive"), but its relation to vaginal carcinoma in the offspring of mothers who took the drug during pregnancy raises doubts about the advisability of its use in any woman of reproductive age. An antiemetic medication may be given with the stilbestrol to minimize the nausea and vomiting. The availability of abortion in the event that the patient who takes these drugs is already pregnant reduces the hazard.

Several steroidal estrogens, none of which has yet been shown to be associated with vaginal or cervical carcinoma, also are effective. Suggested regimens include ethinyl estradiol, 2.5 mg twice a day; estrone, 5 mg twice a day; and conjugated estrogens, 10 mg twice a day. The steroids have not yet been approved by the FDA for use as postcoital contraceptives. Pregnancy can be prevented also by the insertion of a copper intrauterine device within five days of coitus at midcycle. This method has the advantage of providing continued contraception.

Among the experimental techniques, several antizygotic agents have been tested. These drugs are toxic, however, and the differences between abortifacient and teratogenic dosages are small. Again, perhaps the ready availability of abortion may lead to wider use of this class of drugs.

Male chemosterilants are also under investigation. These drugs may suppress spermatogenesis but they are generally toxic, resulting in a decrease in libido and in production of androgens. Some of these drugs have an antabuse effect.

Reversible occlusion of the oviduct has been attempted with drugs such as quinacrine. The quinacrine block may be reversed by estrogen as well as other drugs.

Some but not all recent evidence suggests that prostaglandins may be effective contraceptives or early abortifacients. The mechanism of action of these compounds and their role in population control, however, remain to be elucidated. The principal problem with the presently available prostaglandins is their widespread systemic effects.

A logical approach to contraception is the development of inhibitors to the gonadotropic releasing hormones. Unlike the oral contraceptives, these hormones have a highly localized site of action. An inhibitor to the gonadotropin releasing hormone (GnRH), for example, would specifically inhibit ovulation or spermatogenesis. These compounds are effective in nanogram doses.

The immunologic control of pregnancy has much to commend it theoretically, but has not yet reached the stage of clinical application to human reproduction. Antibodies to the β-subunit of hCG seem to provide a logical means of preventing pregnancy, but the dual problems of reversibility and adverse effects on tissues other than trophoblast remain to be overcome.

Sterilization

Sterilization, a *permanent* form of *contraception,* is an important adjunct to traditional contraception and abortion. It appears to be *more popular* today, probably because of changing personal and societal values. In about one of every five married white couples in the United States between the ages of 20 and 40, a sterilizing procedure has been performed on one of the partners. As of 1978, sterilization has overtaken oral contraception in this group as the most commonly employed means of preventing pregnancy. The pregnancy rate, depending on the technique employed, is between 0.1 and 0.5.

Because of recent changes in attitude, sterilization of the *male* has become much more acceptable. The possibility of *sperm banking* may have added further impetus to male sterilization.

When abortions were permitted for medical reasons only, sterilization was often performed at the time of abortion, presumably because the reason for the abortion was also a reason for preventing further pregnancies. In the case of elective abortions, sterilization is not necessarily indicated.

The major techniques of *female* sterilization involve *ligation* or *resection* of the *oviduct*. The principal forms of tubal sterilization are immediate *postpartum* resection, *laparoscopic* sterilization, and *vaginal* or *abdominal* tubal procedures in the *nonpuerperal* state.

There are several advantages to *postpartum* sterilization: the procedure can be performed in 10 to 20 minutes under the *same anesthetic* that is used for delivery; a *small* abdominal *incision* is sufficient; the additional *cost* to the patient and the additional length of hospitalization are *not* significantly *increased;* and the likelihood of *failure* and *complications* is *small*. The procedure must, however, be discussed with the patient before labor and the possibility that the child may not be of the desired sex or may not survive must be considered.

Laparoscopic sterilization involves induction of a *pneumoperitoneum* (p. 131) and cauterization and partial resection of the tube. Its advantages include a *short hospitalization,* which varies from 8 to 24 hours, a very *small* point of *entry* into the abdomen, and relatively *few complications.* It is not, however, quite so effective as sterilization through a formal laparotomy and it may involve *injury* to neighboring abdominal *viscera.* Several techniques have been devised recently to reduce the likelihood of thermal and electrical injuries during laparoscopy: the *bipolar* method, the Yoon (Falope) *ring,* and the Hulka *clip.* Contraindications to laparoscopic sterilization include abdominal scars, adhesions, hernias, and peritonitis.

An alternative to laparoscopy is *minilaparotomy.* The tubal resection is carried out through a small suprapubic incision. Although the technique is inappropriate for obese women, it requires no elaborate equipment and is therefore more readily applicable to developing countries.

Nonpuerperal sterilization may be performed through the abdominal route (*laparotomy*) or through the vagina (*colpotomy*). Formal laparotomy provides excellent access and visualization with a very high rate of success, but it entails a stay in the hospital of four to seven days, a relatively high cost, and a sizable abdominal scar. Vaginal tubal ligation or resection is performed through an incision in the posterior cul-de-sac. Its advantages are the absence of an abdominal scar and a short hospital stay. Disadvantages include increased difficulty in exposure and identification of the tubes. Postoperative complications including abscesses are somewhat more common than with abdominal procedures. A current or recent pregnancy is a contraindication to the vaginal route. Pelvic adhesions are a relative contraindication.

Hysterectomy, abdominal or vaginal, provides *virtually complete protection* against subsequent pregnancy. It may be performed in conjunction with a cesarean section. It is a *more extensive procedure* than a tubal resection and is associated with a longer hospitalization and a higher incidence of postoperative complications such as hemorrhage, infection, and injury to the urinary tract. In addition to terminating fertility it re-

moves a functionless organ and prevents carcinoma of the corpus or cervix.

Hysterectomy terminates menses, which may be an advantage or a disadvantage, depending on the patient's attitude. Despite the prophylactic value of hysterectomy it probably cannot be justified as a routine alternative to tubal sterilization. It appears most logical when sterilization is to be performed in a patient with uterine disease such as myomas or cervical dysplasia. Even though 10% of women may have gynecologic disease that requires surgical operation after tubal sterilization, the complications of hysterectomy justify the procedure only when there is a reason in addition to termination of childbearing potential or when there are religious objections to tubal sterilization.

The most serious complications of tubal ligation or resection are pulmonary emboli and ectopic pregnancy. A principal technique of tubal resection is the Pomeroy operation, in which the tube is not crushed, an absorbable suture is used, and the knuckle of ligated tube is resected. The failure rate of a properly performed Pomeroy sterilization should not exceed 0.5%. The reversibility of tubal sterilizations varies between 10 and 40%, depending on the procedure used. Techniques involving fimbriectomy and electrocoagulation are less amenable to reversal than are properly performed Pomeroy operations.

In techniques such as the Madlener operation the tube is crushed and ligated with a nonabsorbable suture and the knuckle is not resected. The failure rate of this procedure is considerably higher than that of the Pomeroy operation.

A somewhat more complicated technique with a very high rate of success is the Irving sterilization. In this operation the proximal end of the tube is buried in a tunnel within the myometrium and the distal end is often buried between the leaves of the broad ligament.

Hysteroscopy, a promising endoscopic technique, permits transvaginal cauterization of the uterine ostia of the fallopian tubes. A potentially reversible hysteroscopic technique involves delivery of a plug of methylcyanoacrylate (MCA) into the uterine ostia of the oviducts. The rapid polymerization of the compound prevents spillage into the peritoneal cavity.

Cryosurgical ablation of the endometrium or destruction of the uterotubal junctions is another new technique that has achieved promising results.

The most popular form of male sterilization is *vasectomy.* This procedure involves bilateral scrotal incisions, or occasionally a single midline incision, and division of each ductus deferens. Its advantages are *rapidity, inexpensiveness,* and the possibility of accomplishment in the *office* with only *local anesthesia.* There is no demonstrable effect on production of androgens, libido, or sexual performance. Disadvantages are the fear of impotence by the male and the obvious but crucial fact that the female partner may still become pregnant. Several techniques of reversible male sterilization involving insertion of a removable device into the vas are currently under investigation.

The ejaculate must be shown to be free of spermatozoa on two successive occasions before reliance can be placed on the method for complete contraception. This procedure is reversible in less than 50% of cases. Granulomas that occasionally follow section of the ductus deferens have not caused serious clinical problems. Preliminary reports of autoimmune disease resulting from vasectomy have not been substantiated. The patient must be informed that the long-range viability of banked frozen sperm has not been demonstrated. The potential patient who agrees to vasectomy only on condition of a guarantee that a sample of his banked semen will retain its potential for fertilization and that the procedure is reversible should be discouraged from undergoing the procedure. He should, instead, be offered the alternative of a temporary form of contraception. Ambivalence about any sterilizing procedure in male or female is best managed by deferring permanent forms of contraception.

The Department of Health, Education, and Welfare has recently promulgated regulations governing nontherapeutic sterilizations paid for by federal funds. It has imposed a moratorium on sterilization of minors and mentally incompetent men and women. Furthermore, it has required a greatly detailed informed consent that lists complications of sterilization and alternatives to the procedure. Until 1979 it required that a period of at least 72 hours elapse between the signing of the consent form and the performance of the procedure. Effective March, 1979, H.E.W. has extended the mandatory period of delay to 30 days for federally funded sterilizations, except in certain cases of premature labor or surgical operations performed as emergencies.

Abortion

Although abortion is *not* recommended as a *primary means* of family planning or population control, it serves as a logical *backup* for failed contraception. Perhaps with ready availability of abortion, contraceptives can be developed that are less than 100% effective but are devoid of the complications of the currently available drugs and devices.

Until 1973 abortion was very closely regulated by statute in most of the states to the extent that a serious medical problem was required to justify the procedure. Circumstances in which abortion is mandatory to save the life of the mother are most unusual. They may include advanced cardiac disease with prior decompensation, severe renal or vascular disease, and carcinoma of the cervix. *Psychiatric* indications for abortion and *fetal indications* such as prevention of the birth of an infant with structural or biochemical defects have been subject to wide differences of interpretation by the various states. The most restrictive abortion laws allowed the procedure only to *save the life of the mother.* Other legislatures allowed the procedure to protect the *life or health* of the mother. The more liberal laws defined health, according to the interpretation of the World Health Organization, as including *mental* and *social well-being.* The abortion issue is still debated hotly, largely along religious lines, as a question of *maternal versus fetal rights.*

The status of abortion in the United States was drastically changed by the historic decision of the *United States Supreme Court* on January 22, 1973. The effect of that decision was to strengthen the female's rights, to emancipate the nation from the constraints imposed by the viewpoint of a minority, and to widen the scope of family planning activities. The Supreme Court's decision was influenced by the finding that the fetus has no constitutional rights and that neither biologists, theologians, or legal scholars could agree when life begins. All state laws must now be consistent with the ruling of the Supreme Court, which essentially leaves decisions about abortion in the *first trimester* of pregnancy to the *patient* and her *doctor* without any regulation or interference by the State. For the period from the *end of the first* trimester to approximately the *end of the second* trimester, the State in promoting its interest in the health of the mother may *regulate* but *not prohibit* abortion for the protection of maternal health. For the stage *subsequent to viability,* at approximately the beginning of the third trimester, the State, in promoting its interest in the potentiality of human life, may *regulate or proscribe* abortion, except where the physician reasonably believes an abortion based on physiologic or psychologic grounds to be necessary for the preservation of the life or health of the mother. To comply fully with the ruling of the Supreme Court the State cannot impose the requirement of a husband's signature, for example, in first-trimester abortions.

In 1977 the Supreme Court ruled that individual states are not required to pay for abortions with Medicaid funds. The effect of this decision, which is currently being challenged, is to deny to poor women a medical service that is available to the wealthy. Through the efforts of a well-organized, well-financed minority, many legislatures have begun attempts to erode the liberal laws governing abortion. Requirements such as spousal and parental consent, though contrary to the Supreme Court ruling of 1973, have recently been legislated in several states. Before the decisions are reversed, however, it is likely that many unwanted pregnancies and septic abortions will result.

Techniques of abortion fall into several main categories: *dilatation* of the cervix followed by sharp *curettage* or evacuation by *suction,* instillation of *solutions* into the *amniotic cavity, hysterotomy,* and *hysterectomy.*

Medicinal induction of abortion is not considered further here. Oxytocin is not effective in the early stages of pregnancy and intravenous and extraamniotic prostaglandins and numerous herbal and folk remedies are insufficiently tested to be recommended as routine abortifacients.

The principal technique for evacuating the uterus *under 12 weeks'* gestational size is curettage, by *sharp curette* or *suction*. Because it is slightly less dangerous and can be performed on larger uteri, the suction technique is more widely used today. Occasionally it is necessary to remove some products of conception by gentle sharp curettage after an attempt at evacuation by suction.

A modification of the suction technique applicable to very early pregnancy involves the insertion of a semirigid *plastic catheter,* with dimensions approximately equal to those of an ordinary drinking straw, through the virtually undilated cervix. Suction may then be applied and products of conception removed. Such techniques performed at the time of the first missed period or earlier have been termed "menstrual regulation" or "*menstrual induction,*" but they are merely early abortions.

Dilatation and curettage or suction require a block or a general anesthetic, but may be performed as an *outpatient procedure* within a hospital or in a facility with immediate access to a hospital for the management of complications. The time required for the surgical procedure and recovery is short. Disadvantages of the procedure are the occasional injury to the cervix during dilatation and the occasional perforation of the uterus, which may require laparotomy. Infection, hemorrhage, and the likelihood of perforation increase with the size of the uterus and decrease with the experience of the operator.

Injections of *intraamniotic solutions* are most effectively performed in a uterus of *16 weeks' gestational* size or greater. Until quite recently it was considered desirable to perform the abortion before 12 weeks' gestation, when a curettage can be performed with minimal danger, or to wait until 16 weeks, when intraamniotic solutions may be instilled. Between 1976 and 1978, several centers have reported successful results with dilation and evacuation of the uterus larger than 12 weeks' gestational size. The data show that in well-trained hands, *midtrimester abortion* (up to 16 gestational weeks) by *suction* may be safer than intraamniotic solutions of prostaglandin or saline. Data from the Center for Disease Control in Atlanta, reported in 1977, indicate fewer maternal deaths associated with saline than with prostaglandin. Before injection of intraamniotic solutions it is advantageous that the *placenta be located* by sonography to avoid fetomaternal hemorrhage. The amniocentesis is then performed, removing 100 to 200 ml of amniotic fluid, which is replaced very slowly by the abortifacient solution. The most commonly used solutions for this purpose are *prostaglandins* and *hypertonic saline* (20 to 23% NaCl). Dextrose (50%) and urea are less commonly used and ethanol is currently under investigation.

Variations in technique include simultaneous intraamniotic instillation of prostaglandin and urea, intraamniotic prostaglandin and intravenous oxytocin, and intraamniotic urea and intravenous oxytocin. The insertion of laminaria tents into the cervical canal the night before abortion reduces the likelihood of damage to the cervix by forcible instrumental dilation or precipitous delivery through an undilated and uneffaced cervix.

Advantages of abortion through injection of intraamniotic solutions include avoidance of instrumental dilatation of the cervix and laparotomy. Abortion usually follows injection of the solutions by *24 to 36 hours.* The procedure is generally considered a failure if abortion has not occurred within 48 hours after injection. In cases of failure the procedure may be repeated, perhaps with the addition of oxytocin, or a hysterotomy may be performed. Injection of hypertonic saline is *contraindicated* in the presence of *cardiovascular* or *renal disease* and is impossible in the presence of *ruptured membranes.* Injection of *dextrose,* although less likely to aggravate cardiorenal disorders, is accompanied by an increased likelihood of *infection.*

The main *complications* of injection of saline result from inadvertent *intravascular* or *intraperitoneal injection.* They include hypernatremia, cardiac arrest, pulmonary edema, hemoglobinuria, encephalopathy, and necrosis of tissues. Occasionally hemorrhage, infection, and retained products of conception may require curettage. Increasing numbers of cases of *defective coagulation* associated with injection of saline are appearing in the obstetric literature. They are probably examples of disseminated intravascular coagulation. Prostaglandins often result in incomplete abortions, which may require completion by curettage. In addition, their use occasionally results in delivery of a living fetus. Intraamniotic solutions are less popular than they were a few years ago.

Ideally, abortions should be *prevented* by effective *contraception;* when unwanted pregnancy requires abortion, the procedure should be done as *early* in pregnancy as possible in the interests of *maternal safety.*

Hysterotomy is occasionally performed for abortion when the uterus is too large to empty by curettage or suction and when intraamniotic solutions are ineffective or medically contraindicated. Disadvantages of hysterotomy include the prolonged hospitalization (5 to 8 days) and the scars in the abdomen and uterus, which may require subsequent delivery by cesarean section.

Abortion may also be effected through *hysterectomy.* The advantages of the procedure include the removal of a potentially or an actually diseased organ and *permanent sterilization.* Disadvantages include the *increased morbidity* associated with hysterectomy in general. The special example of carcinoma of the cervix complicating early pregnancy is best managed by abortion through simultaneous radical hysterectomy and pelvic lymph node dissection or complete radiotherapy. Pregnancy in the patient with cardiac disease may often logically be interrupted by hysterectomy (supracervical or total) rather than hysterotomy.

In February, 1973, the American College of Obstetricians and Gynecologists issued a statement that describes the ideal circumstances for performance of an elective abortion. Abortion should be regarded as a surgical procedure and its performance should require appropriate surgical, anesthetic, and resuscitative equipment. In addition, the diagnosis and duration of pregnancy should be verified. Laboratory procedures should include blood typing and identification of the Rh-type. Any factors or illness that might have a bearing on the anesthesia and any drug sensitivities should be recorded.

Rh immune globulin (p. 104) is often given after abortion to any Rh-negative patient when the father's Rh-type is positive or unknown. It is not necessary to give a full dose of 300 μg, especially in very early abortion, when the extent of feto-maternal hemorrhage is minimal. Postoperative and contraceptive advice should be available. No physician should be required to perform an abortion and no patient should be forced to undergo the procedure. An informed consent should be obtained and the procedure should be performed only by physicians who are qualified to identify and manage the complications that may arise from the procedure. Attempts should be made to provide facilities where abortions can be performed with maximal safety but with minimal disruption of other hospital functions.

UNIT VIII

Human Sexuality

Detailed discussions of human sexuality are beyond the scope of even large textbooks of gynecology, but awareness of the wide range of normal sexual behavior and recognition of common psychosexual problems are requisite to effective gynecologic diagnosis and therapy. The necessity for obtaining a *complete factual history* of sexual habits is discussed in Unit I. The same objectivity should be applied to this area of gynecology as to a discussion of cardiovascular or gastrointestinal function. The criteria of sexuality are enumerated on page 207.

The gynecologist is often the first physician to deal with female sexual inadequacies and is also required to exclude organic causes of sexual dysfunction in his patients. He must be competent to counsel young patients and avert psychosexual neuroses. *Control of conception* is one important facet of sexual counseling, for fear of pregnancy may lead to sexual inadequacy.

The physician requires knowledge of sex-specific differences in the *cycle of sexual response* and the *wide variations* in psychologic attitudes and physical behavior in both sexes. The physician must differentiate *sexual problems* based on *ignorance* from true *sexual neuroses* and *organic diseases*. He must recognize the enormous variety of *cultural mores* and *taboos* and strive to prevent his own sexual inhibitions from interfering with effective rapport with the patient. He must expand his concept of *normal sexual behavior*, which is defined by some experts in the area as including any activity that mutually pleases two consenting adults without causing physical or psychologic harm.

Statistically, an act may be classified as normal if it is practiced without deleterious effects by large numbers of people. In this sense, orogenital activity, masturbation, and in some circumstances, homosexual relations between consenting adults can no longer be classified as aberrations. The physician must help destroy psychologically harmful *sexual myths*. In particular, he must assure his patient that some form of *masturbation* is almost universally practiced at certain times of life and that it serves a useful function in relieving tension. He must also dispel the myths about the value, or indeed the existence, of specific *aphrodisiacs*. It is important that he *distinguish love from sex* and explain the differences to his patients.

The physician should be familiar with the basic *Freudian concepts* and recognize the need for psychiatric referral. He should be aware of *changing patterns of sexuality* and the sexual readjustments by men and women that are created by female liberation, the abolition of the double sexual standard, and the active role assumed by women in sexual encounters. The physician must be able to explain to the patient the *changes in sexual response* after major gynecologic operations and during the prenatal course and post partum. He should discourage unnecessary restriction of sexual activity in pregnancy that is based on unfounded fears of injuring the fetus or inducing prematurity. He should explain that the woman's libido may be increased or decreased during her pregnancy, whereas the male's is likely to remain unchanged. The physician should understand that *sexual activity* and sexual problems may involve patients of *advanced age*.

Sexual counseling requires time and patience. The first visit is often devoted simply to establishing confidence of the patients in the physician. Successful treatment requires a careful sexual history obtained independently from each partner. Difficult problems should be referred to expert sexual counselors, often a team comprising a gynecologist and a psychologist. Deep-seated neuroses should be referred to a psychiatrist.

The *frequency* of sexual activity varies enormously within any age group, although in general, frequency decreases with age. *Libido in women* increases between the early twenties and the middle thirties. *In men* libido is greatest in the late teens, decreasing notably in the late twenties. In both sexes libido may continue into advanced years. It is affected throughout life by general mental health, depression, and anxiety. It is influenced also by chronic alcoholism and by drugs such as morphine, heroin, and LSD.

Human Sexual Response

Human sexual response is basically *similar in both sexes*. Sexual stimulation leads to *vascular engorgement, muscular tension,* and their physiologic consequences. The four phases of sexual response described by Masters and Johnson are *excitement, plateau, orgasm,* and *resolution.* The details are given on pages 254 through 257. The excitement phase is the longest. It may be induced by somatic or psychogenic stimuli and delayed or interrupted voluntarily.

Whereas the female may have *multiple orgasms* in rapid succession, the male undergoes a *refractory period* of five to 30 minutes, during which orgasm cannot be achieved by any means. Ordinarily orgasm in the male is reached faster and more directly than in the female, in whom physical contact appears to be a less significant erotogenic factor. The feeling that the female is desired may in itself lead to heightened sexual response. The intensity of the female reaction may depend upon amount and type of foreplay. The physician should advise against attempts to attain simultaneous orgasms in both partners, for such a result is neither common nor necessarily desirable. He should also refute the concept of the superiority of vaginal over clitoral orgasm, since, despite Freud's teaching, the two means of stimulation produce identical orgasms. Direct contact with the clitoris is not usually achieved during intercourse in the "missionary position" (man over woman), since the clitoris normally retracts under the symphysis. Effective stimulation of the clitoris is more directly achieved by digital manipulation.

Another myth concerns the advantage of the large over the small penis as an effective organ of copulation, for there is relatively little difference in size among erect penises; nor does circumcision increase or decrease sensation or delay ejaculation. Most important, the physician should recognize that *sexual incompatibilities* are usually *psychogenic* rather than physical. He should identify serious psychosexual disorders and obtain psychiatric consultation at the first opportunity.

The details of human sexual response have been described in the writings of Masters and Johnson. In general, there is notable similarity in the genital and extragenital responses in both men and women during excitement, plateau, orgasm, and resolution.

During the excitement phase in women there is tumescence of the glans of the clitoris, vasocongestion, and increase in diameter and length of the shaft. The vagina provides lubrication within 10 to 30 seconds of stimulation and the vaginal tube expands and assumes a darker purplish hue. The uterus is partially elevated and the corpus becomes irritable. The labia majora in the nullipara undergo flattening, separation, and anterolateral elevation away from the vaginal outlet; in the multipara vasocongestion, increase in diameter, and slight movement away from the midline occur. The labia minora undergo slight thickening and expansion.

In the plateau phase the clitoris retracts under the symphysis. The vagina forms an orgasmic platform at its outer third and undergoes further increase in width and depth. Corpus and cervix are fully elevated and there is further increase in irritability of the corpus. The labia majora in the nullipara are severely engorged; in the multipara further vasocongestion occurs. The labia minora undergo a striking change in color from bright red to deep wine, indicating impending orgasm. At this stage Bartholin's glands secrete a drop or two of mucoid material.

At orgasm, contractions of the orgasmic platform in the vagina are noted at intervals of 0.8 seconds, recurring 6 to 12 times. The uterus undergoes contractions, the extent of which parallels the intensity of the orgasm. In the multipara there may be up to a 50% increase in uterine size.

During the phase of resolution the clitoris returns to its normal position. Five to 10 seconds after orgasm the platform ceases to contract and undergoes rapid detumescence. The vaginal walls relax and their normal color returns within 10 to 15 minutes. The uterus returns to its normal position, but the external os continues to gape for about 20 to 30 minutes. In the nullipara, the labia majora return to their normal thickness and midline position; in the multipara, the labial vasocongestion disappears. The labia minora change color from bright red to light pink within 15 seconds and their size decreases.

In addition, there are numerous extragenital reactions during the various phases of female sexual response. During excitement several changes occur in the breasts. The nipples become erect and increase in size; concomitant tumescence of the areolae occurs. A maculopapular rash (sex flush) develops late in the phase of excitement, beginning over the epigastrium and spreading over the breasts. Myotonia, both voluntary and involuntary, increases. Tachycardia parallels the degree of sexual tension.

During the plateau phase the nipples become turgid. The breasts increase further in size and the areolae undergo further erection. The sex flush is better developed and myotonia increases, accompanied by spastic contractions. Tachycardia increases to as high as 175/minute, accompanied by increases in systolic and diastolic blood pressures of 20 to 60 and 10 to 20 mm Hg, respectively.

At the time of orgasm the sex flush parallels the intensity of the reaction. Myotonia is maximal, with loss of voluntary control, accompanied by involuntary contractions of the rectal sphincter. The respiratory rate increases to as high as 40/minute and tachycardia increases to between 110 and 180/minute. Blood pressure rises about 30 to 50 mm Hg systolic and 20 to 40 mm Hg diastolic.

During resolution rapid detumescence of the nipples and areolae occurs. The decrease in volume of the breasts is slower. The sex flush disappears rapidly in the reverse order in which it appeared. Myotonia rarely continues for more than five minutes after orgasm. Hyperventilation and tachycardia return rapidly to normal. A widespread film of perspiration appears, unrelated to the extent of physical activity.

In the male, the genital and extragenital reactions are similar to those just described in the female. During excitement the most obvious event is the rapid erection of the penis. Erection may be lost and regained or inhibited by numerous stimuli during this phase. There is tensing and thickening of the scrotal skin and elevation of the sac. The testes are elevated as a result of shortening of the spermatic cords.

During the plateau phase the penis undergoes an increase in circumference at the coronal ridge and possibly a change in color of the corona. The testes are said to undergo an enlargement of 50% over their nonstimulated state. Full elevation of the testes indicates impending ejaculation. Cowper's glands provide a preejaculatory emission of a few drops of fluid containing numerous active spermatozoa.

At orgasm the penis undergoes contraction along the entire length of the penile urethra. The contractions start at intervals of 0.8 seconds. After the first three or four contractions, the expulsive force is reduced.

During resolution the penis undergoes detumescence in two stages, a rapid and a slow. The scrotum rapidly loses its congestion and its normal folds reappear. The testes return to normal size and position.

The male also undergoes certain extragenital reactions. In excitement there is occasional erection of the nipples, myotonia (including voluntary and involuntary components), and tachycardia and hypertension in proportion to the degree of sexual tension.

During the plateau phase, an inconsistent further increase in erection of the nipples occurs. A maculopapular rash develops late in this phase. The rash originates over the epigastrium and spreads to the chest wall, neck, forehead, and other locations. Myotonia is characterized by a further increase in voluntary and involuntary components. Hyperventilation occurs late in this phase, and tachycardia may range between 100 and 175/minute, with an increase in blood pressure from 20 to 80 mm Hg systolic and 10 to 40 diastolic.

At orgasm, a well-developed sex flush is seen in about 25% of men. Myotonia is characterized by loss of voluntary control and by involuntary contractions and spasm. The rectal sphincter undergoes contractions occurring at intervals of 0.8/second and the respiratory rate may rise to as high as 40/minute. Tachycardia ranges from 110 to 180, and a rise in blood pressure of 40 to 100 systolic and 20 to 50 diastolic occurs.

During resolution there is involution of erection of the nipples and rapid disappearance of the sex flush in reverse order of its appearance. Myotonia disappears within five minutes after the end of orgasm. The increased blood pressure, heart rate, and respiratory rate return to normal. Perspiration in the male is inconsistent and involuntary and is usually confined to the palms and soles.

Common Sexual Complaints

Sexual dysfunction may result from disorders of sexual *desire* or *arousal*. Education and counseling are of great benefit in simple cases of ignorance of sexual function. Disorders of female arousal are sometimes effectively treated by so-called *sensate focus* exercises. With this technique the male is asked to defer orgasm as he proceeds through three stages of sexual activity. The first stage avoids contact with either the female genitalia or breasts. In the second stage the breasts are stimulated. In the third stage coitus is permitted. The woman assumes a superior position, which increases her control of the coital act. She initiates intercourse and thrusts slowly while contracting her pubococcygeal muscles.

Orgasmic dysfunction may be treated by teaching the woman how to *masturbate*. If manual stimulation of the clitoris and breasts is ineffective, she may use a vibrator. Sexual reeducation in this disorder involves the woman's deferring coitus until she is close to orgasm, use of fantasy, contraction of the perineal and abdominal muscles, use of the stop-start technique, adjunctive stimulation of the clitoris during coitus, and rapid thrusting by the woman when she feels an impending orgasm.

Pelvic congestion is a vague syndrome of neurovascular origin. It may be a manifestation of *psychosexual conflict,* fear of pregnancy, inadequate sexual response, or failure of orgasm. The venous channels of the pelvis are congested and the uterosacral ligaments are indurated. Deep pelvic pain increases just before menses and dyspareunia is common. Diagnosis is suggested by *multiple complaints* in an unusually *tense patient.* The uterus is often retroverted and enlarged to the size of a 10 weeks' gestation. Differential diagnosis includes endometriosis (p. 153) and chronic pelvic inflammatory disease (p. 145). In the pelvic congestion syndrome, unlike endometriosis, the *tense ligaments* seem to *disappear under anesthesia*. Treatment may include *tranquilizers, psychotherapy,* and *adrenergic blocking agents.*

Dyspareunia, painful or otherwise unsatisfactory intercourse, may result from organic causes such as atrophy of the introitus, scars, or severe vaginitis. Additional common causes include endometriosis of the uterosacral ligaments, the pelvic congestion syndrome, and purely psychogenic factors.

Vaginismus is painful spasm of the vagina, sufficient to prevent satisfactory coitus. The pelvic muscles are spastic and penetration may be prevented. It may be caused by repugnance to the sexual act and is almost always psychogenic. Use of progressively larger dilators is occasionally effective.

Frigidity, or sexual coldness, is lack of libido or desire for the sexual act. It should be differentiated from lack of orgasm. Permanent frigidity is psychosexual, perhaps representing subconscious repression. Women with frigidity may achieve orgasm by masturbation.

Nymphomania is defined as extreme eroticism or sexual desire in women. It corresponds to satyriasis in men. These are poor terms because eroticism is most difficult to quantitate.

Premature ejaculation is defined as failure to delay ejaculation for 30 seconds after penetration. It is a very common complaint, which only in its severe or chronic form may be termed a psychosexual disorder. A technique in which the penis is squeezed by the partner is frequently recommended to delay ejaculation.

Impotence is failure to achieve and maintain an erection during coitus. It is primarily a psychologic problem, in which fear of failure to perform well sexually may create a vicious cycle.

APPENDIX

An Outline of Obstetric and Gynecologic Emergencies*

*Although this material is presented in outline rather than narrative style, it should be considered required (Class I) information. Cross-references to the text proper are included.

I. General Principles

A. Most patients with obstetric or gynecologic emergencies present with low abdominal pain, uterine bleeding, or both. In women of any age, therefore, such pain or bleeding should suggest a gynecologic disorder.

B. If the patient is of reproductive age, an obstetric complication must be considered in addition.

C. Although pregnancy is normally a physiologic process, certain hemorrhagic disorders of the third trimester are the most serious and rapidly fatal accidents in the field of medicine. In general, obstetric-gynecologic consultation should be obtained immediately while emergency measures are being instituted.

II. Ectopic Pregnancy (p. 80)

A. Because rupture of a pregnant oviduct may lead to maternal hemorrhage and death, this diagnosis always must be considered in a woman of childbearing age with vaginal bleeding and abdominal pain.

B. In the vast majority of cases the ectopic pregnancy involves the oviduct, and because this disorder masquerades in many guises, it must be considered seriously in any woman with an atypical first-trimester pregnancy.

C. Classically, the triad of menstrual disturbance, vaginal bleeding, and an adnexal mass is described, but any or all of these features may be lacking. Amenorrhea helps make the diagnosis of pregnancy, but often some other change in the menses or none at all is reported.

D. Instead of frank vaginal bleeding there may be merely sanguineous or brownish discharge.

E. If the pregnant tube has ruptured, syncope, a fall in blood pressure, a rise in pulse rate, and a low hematocrit may supervene. The leukocyte count is usually normal or only slightly elevated.

F. On pelvic examination pain on motion of the cervix is usually detected. The uterus is often enlarged to the size of a six to eight weeks' intrauterine pregnancy, and a boggy mass may be felt in the adnexa on one side.

G. In the face of signs of rupture of the tube with intraperitoneal hemorrhage, blood must be typed and crossmatched immediately, an intravenous infusion begun through a large-bore needle (18-gauge or larger), gynecologic consultation obtained immediately, and the operating room alerted to the likelihood of an emergency laparotomy.

H. Immunologic tests for pregnancy are usually unrewarding and often misleading. Attempts at confirmation of hemoperitoneum by culdocentesis should not delay gynecologic consultation and admittance of the patient. The rate of false-negative and false-positive taps, furthermore, may be high.

III. Pelvic Inflammatory Disease (p. 143)

A. The patient with acute pelvic inflammatory disease often presents with low abdominal pain and fever. She frequently dates the onset of symptoms from her last menstrual period.

B. The abdominal pain is usually bilateral, beginning in the lower quadrants but later becoming generalized.

C. Nausea is common but vomiting is not ordinarily an early sign.

D. The fever and leukocyte count are usually higher in pelvic inflammatory disease (P.I.D.) than in acute appendicitis or ectopic pregnancy, the two surgical conditions with which P.I.D. is most commonly confused.

E. The early phase of acute pelvic inflammatory disease is usually unaccompanied by signs and symptoms referable to the gastrointestinal tract.

F. When such signs appear, attention must be directed to appendicitis, diverticulitis, chronic pelvic inflammatory disease with intestinal obstruction, and rupture of a tubo-ovarian abscess.

G. Acute P.I.D. is often accompanied by vaginal discharge, but the blood pressure is unchanged and the pulse rate is usually elevated only in proportion to the fever.

H. The hematocrit remains stable and the leukocyte count ranges from about normal to well over 15,000. Shock is uncommon except with rupture of an abscess, an abdominal catastrophe that requires immediate admittance of the patient and laparotomy as a life-saving procedure.

I. Unlike ectopic pregnancy with which it is easily confused, pelvic inflammatory disease is unaccompanied by signs of pregnancy. In acute P.I.D. no adnexal masses are usually palpable, but pain on motion of the cervix is frequently elicited before unequivocal signs of pelvic peritonitis are detected.

J. If the slightest doubt about the possibility of ectopic pregnancy or acute appendicitis remains, the patient must be admitted. In any case gynecologic consultation must be obtained without delay.

K. In certain cases of mild acute pelvic inflammatory disease the gynecologic consultant may decide to discharge the patient on antibiotic therapy, but reexamination within 24 to 48 hours is mandatory to confirm the diagnosis and evaluate success of medical treatment. The patient must be cautioned to return promptly if pain increases or any additional signs or symptoms occur.

IV. Differential Diagnosis of Lower Abdominal Pain

A. *Appendicitis*

1. The pain begins in the upper abdomen. If pain appears lower in the abdomen it is often most severe in the right lower quadrant.
2. Unlike the pain of gynecologic disorders, that of appendicitis ordinarily bears no relation to the menses.
3. In appendicitis, nausea and vomiting occur earlier than in ectopic pregnancy and P.I.D.
4. In both acute appendicitis and ectopic pregnancy, fever and leukocytosis are usually less pronounced than in pelvic inflammatory disease. In acute appendicitis the leukocyte count is commonly in the range of 12,000 to 15,000 unless generalized peritonitis supervenes. In acute pelvic inflammatory disease it is frequently above 15,000.
5. Point tenderness is more common in appendicitis, whereas with pelvic inflammatory disease (acute salpingitis) associated peritonitis is usually detected earlier.

B. *Torsion of an ovarian tumor,* like ectopic pregnancy, may be associated with an adnexal mass and pain on motion of the cervix.

C. A *hemorrhagic corpus luteum cyst* may simulate ectopic pregnancy quite closely, with respect to slight enlargement of the uterus, adnexal mass, pain on motion of the cervix, amenorrhea, and even signs of intraperitoneal hemorrhage. In all such difficult diagnostic problems, gynecologic consultation and, usually, admittance of the patient are mandatory.

V. Abortion (p. 76)

A. A pregnant patient with vaginal bleeding during the first 20 weeks of pregnancy, by definition, has a *threatened* abortion.

B. The bleeding is occasionally accompanied by mild abdominal cramps or back pain.

C. Ordinarily no treatment, except possibly bedrest, is required, but because threatened abortion may mimic ectopic pregnancy with respect to amenorrhea, vaginal bleeding, and uterine enlargement, and even an adnexal mass (corpus luteum of pregnancy), the patient should be seen by a gynecologic consultant before discharge from the emergency room.

D. The gynecologist will inspect her cervix and vagina through a speculum with a good light to rule out traumatic or neoplastic causes of the bleeding unrelated to abortion.

E. If no extrauterine cause for the bleeding is found and the cervix is closed with the membranes intact, the gynecologist may choose to care for the patient on an outpatient basis; if so, he will provide her with strict instructions to return if bleeding becomes copious or is accompanied by severe cramps.

F. At this point, the cervix usually begins to dilate and the abortion becomes *imminent*. When the membranes rupture, the abortion becomes *inevitable*. These two varieties of abortion are best managed in the hospital.

G. If on the first visit to the emergency service the patient has severe bleeding and a low hematocrit, blood should be typed and crossmatched without delay while gynecologic consultation is called and rapid admittance procedures are initiated.

H. If any of the products of conception are passed, an *incomplete* abortion results. The condition is usually treated by complete evacuation of the uterus by suction or sharp curettage.

I. Any aborting patient with signs of infection or shock, particularly if a history of instrumental induction is elicited, must be admitted. The sequelae of infected abortion, which may be life-threatening, include septic shock, often caused by endotoxins produced by gram-negative organisms and less frequently by clostridial exotoxins.

J. The diagnosis of *septic shock* calls for immediate gynecologic consultation and admittance. Blood must be typed and crossmatched, an intravenous infusion started through a large-gauge needle, and cultures of the cervix obtained.

K. Lacerations of the cervix and vagina and perforation of the uterus must be ruled out as quickly as possible.

L. An upright roentgenogram of the abdomen should be obtained to rule out perforation, which may be suggested by air under the diaphragm.

M. Patients with endotoxic shock often arrive in the emergency room critically ill, with hypotension and oliguria. In these cases a bladder catheter should be inserted promptly to monitor urinary output.

N. Consultation with the renal team is urgent at this point, for prognosis depends on removal from the uterus of as much infected material as possible as well as management of the renal tubular damage.

O. In clostridial infections, hemolysis may be superimposed on oliguria and hypotension. No time should be wasted in trying to obtain a history of criminal interference, for patients will often die before admitting to abortion. Instead, rapid admittance and coordinated activity of gynecologist and nephrologist may be life-saving measures.

P. *Intraamniotic hypertonic saline* is still occasionally used to interrupt midtrimester pregnancies. Although it is safer to keep the patient in the hospital until the abortion is completed, she is occasionally discharged with instructions to return at the onset of uterine cramps. The intraamniotic injection may produce hypernatremia, with resulting cardiac arrest, hemoglobinuria, or encephalopathy.

VI. Ovarian Cysts (p. 14)

A. Although most large ovarian tumors do not undergo torsion to produce gynecologic emergencies, patients with very large abdominal masses may appear in the emergency room in respiratory distress. In such cases it is desirable to differentiate a large ovarian cystic mass from *ascites*.

B. With ovarian cysts, the abdomen is rounded below and flat above. There is seldom shifting dullness.

C. On percussion, tympany is elicited in the flanks and near the xiphoid, and dullness around the umbilicus. The intestines are displaced laterally and superiorly.

D. With ascites, the abdomen is more nearly symmetric. Shifting dullness is elicited, and the flanks and xiphoid region are dull to percussion, with tympany around the umbilicus.

E. Inserting a trochar or heavy needle into the abdomen of a woman in the emergency room in order to differentiate these two conditions is both dangerous and unwise. Instead, consultations with the gynecologist and other appropriate specialists must be obtained without delay.

VII. Rape

A. Women who have been or claim to have been raped may appear in the emergency room, often with a police escort, for examination and possible treatment.

B. The physician's duty at such times is to record the history as accurately as possible, preferably in the patient's own words, and to record objectively the physical findings.

C. The emergency room physician may describe the condition of the clothing and record whether there are bruises or lacerations on the patient's body.

D. The gynecologic consultant should perform an examination of the lower abdomen, buttocks, and external genitalia to record injuries. The throat and rectum should be examined as well. He next examines the condition of the hymen.

E. A speculum should be inserted, if possible, to expose the cervix, and a specimen of fluid from the vagina should be examined to detect spermatozoa or acid phosphatase.

F. The possibility of venereal disease and pregnancy should be discussed with the patient by the gynecologist and appropriate treatment instituted. If the patient is not already pregnant, stilbestrol (50 mg/day × 5 days), or possibly a copper-containing IUD, may be given as a postcoital contraceptive (p. 238). A counselor should be available to minimize the likelihood of adverse psychological sequelae.

VIII. Obstetric Emergencies

A. Any pregnant patient with a medical emergency should be seen promptly by the obstetric consultant. Certain complications, such as cardiac disease and diabetes, are modified by the pregnancy to the extent that expert obstetric consultation is mandatory.

B. In cases of doubt, it is preferable to admit the patient to the obstetric service and obtain appropriate medical consultations there.

C. Because most drugs used to treat maternal diseases cross the placenta and affect the fetus, it is advisable to obtain obstetric consultation before administering any drug, even aspirin, to a pregnant patient (p. 48).

D. A frequently encountered and inappropriately treated medical complication of obstetrics is acute *pyelonephritis,* the most common renal disease in pregnancy (p. 113).

   1. Because of the varied effects of chemotherapeutic agents on mother and fetus at different stages of pregnancy, it is good practice to obtain obstetric consultation in the case of any pregnant patient with flank pain.
   2. Pyelonephritis in pregnancy may be a serious disease that requires hospitalization and prolonged chemotherapy and follow-up. The patient should not be discharged from the emergency room with a supply of antibacterial drugs without preliminary consultation with the obstetrician.

IX. Placenta Previa (p. 86)

A. Although some patients who bleed in the third trimester may be having merely heavy show signaling labor, others may have placenta previa or abruptio placentae, both of which may be life-threatening to the mother if managed with insufficient speed and skill. For this reason all patients who bleed late in pregnancy must have the benefit of immediate obstetric consultation in the emergency room.

B. No vaginal or rectal examinations may be performed on a patient with third trimester bleeding in any circumstances. If the patient has placenta previa, a vaginal or rectal examination may provoke torrential or fatal hemorrhage.

C. The main duty of the emergency room physician is to call the obstetric consultant immediately and prepare for emergency admittance. He should draw blood for typing and crossmatching and insert a large-bore needle for intravenous infusions or blood transfusions.

D. The patient with painless, bright red bleeding in the third trimester must be considered to have placenta previa until proved otherwise.

E. The obstetric consultant may elect to perform a gentle speculum examination to rule out local traumatic or neoplastic causes of the bleeding, but digital examination may be performed only in the operating room with immediate preparations for cesarean section. Definitive diagnosis and management of placenta previa are exclusively inpatient procedures.

X. Abruptio Placentae (p. 88)

A. This complication is classically characterized by vaginal bleeding in the third trimester, often with hypertonic painful uterine contractions; however, pain may be absent and bleeding may be concealed.

B. Fetal death, as witnessed by absence of fetal heart tones, may have occurred by the time the patient reaches the emergency room. As with suspected placenta previa, no attempts at definitive diagnosis should be made in the emergency room.

C. Obstetric consultation should be obtained and admittance procedures begun.

D. An intravenous infusion is started through a large-bore needle and blood is drawn for typing and crossmatching. The blood should be observed for clotting, for some cases of severe abruptio placentae are complicated by hypofibrinogenemia.

E. Additional complications of severe abruption include maternal shock, oliguria, and renal tubular damage.

XI. Eclampsia (p. 99)

A. Eclampsia is a life-endangering condition characterized by convulsions superimposed on the classic triad (preeclampsia) of hypertension, edema, and proteinuria.

B. Any pregnant patient with convulsions must be assumed to have eclampsia until proved otherwise. For this reason immediate obstetric consultation and preparations for admittance of the patient to the obstetric service are mandatory.

C. Emergency treatment of epilepsy incorrectly diagnosed as eclampsia is innocuous to the patient, but if the eclampsia is erroneously managed as epilepsy the patient may continue to convulse and die.

D. A pregnant patient with convulsions must not be admitted to the neurologic or neurosurgical service for diagnosis but only to the obstetric floor. If she later proves to have epilepsy or some other form of noneclamptic convulsions, she may then be transferred to the appropriate service.

E. While waiting for the obstetric consultant, the emergency room physician may insert a catheter into the bladder to monitor the urinary output and to test the urine for glucose and albumin.

F. The possibility of insulin overdosage should be considered in any patient with a history of diabetes. Blood pressure should be recorded and a salt-free intravenous infusion begun.

G. The emergency room physician may give one dose of anticonvulsant medication and insert a padded tongue blade into the patient's mouth if her reflexes are still hyperactive or if she is postictal. The obstetric consultant may then begin magnesium sulfate therapy while proceeding with further diagnostic workup.

XII. Premature Rupture of the Membranes (p. 85)

A. Rupture of the membranes before the onset of labor is often managed aggressively. Any patient in whom leakage of amniotic fluid from the vagina can be demonstrated should be admitted to the obstetric service.

B. In general, all patients with signs of intrauterine infection will be delivered promptly despite the degree of fetal maturity.
C. Afebrile patients will be managed on the obstetric service according to the maturity of the fetus.
D. Any patient who complains of leakage of fluid (amniotic or otherwise) from the vagina must be seen by an obstetric consultant before she is discharged.

XIII. Amniotic Fluid Embolism (p. 90)

A. This uncommon but often fatal complication usually occurs intrapartum or immediately postpartum and is therefore rarely seen in the emergency room except in patients who arrive in the wake of a precipitate delivery.
B. The patient may present with dyspnea, cyanosis, shock, and possibly pulmonary edema.
C. This dangerous combination of signs and symptoms is usually fatal in its severe form. Obstetric and anesthesiologic consultants should be called immediately to the emergency service.
D. Treatment of patients surviving the initial insult comprises oxygen, fluid infusion or blood transfusion, and appropriate measures, for example heparin, for those who develop a clotting defect.

XIV. Thrombophlebitis (p. 119)

A. Postpartum thrombophlebitis is a potentially serious complication that should be treated vigorously on an inpatient basis, because of the possibly associated pulmonary embolism. Obstetric consultation should be obtained promptly.
B. The patient's disease is best managed in the hospital by a team of obstetric and medical consultants.
C. In nonpregnant or nonpuerperal women presenting with what appears to be thrombophlebitis or pulmonary embolism, a history of hormonal contraceptives may provide valuable etiologic clues.
D. A history of steroidal contraception should also be obtained in otherwise healthy young women who present with sudden loss of vision, coronary thrombosis, or cerebral accidents.

Index